Dementia

NEUROLOGY IN PRACTICE:

SERIES EDITORS: ROBERT A. GROSS, DEPARTMENT OF NEUROLOGY, UNIVERSITY
OF ROCHESTER MEDICAL CENTER, ROCHESTER, NY, USA

JONATHAN W. MINK, DEPARTMENT OF NEUROLOGY, UNIVERSITY OF ROCHESTER
MEDICAL CENTER, ROCHESTER, NY, USA

Dementia

EDITED BY

Joseph F. Quinn, MD

Department of Neurology
Oregon Health and Science University
Portland VA Medical Center
Portland, OR, USA

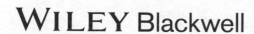

This edition first published 2014, © 2014 by John Wiley & Sons, Ltd

Registered Office
John Wiley & Sons, Ltd, The Atrium, Southern Gate, Chichester, West Sussex, PO19 8SQ, UK

Editorial Offices
9600 Garsington Road, Oxford, OX4 2DQ, UK
The Atrium, Southern Gate, Chichester, West Sussex, PO19 8SQ, UK
111 River Street, Hoboken, NJ 07030-5774, USA

For details of our global editorial offices, for customer services and for information about how to apply for permission to reuse the copyright material in this book please see our website at www.wiley.com/wiley-blackwell.

Library of Congress Cataloging-in-Publication Data

Dementia (Quinn)
  Dementia / edited by Joseph F. Quinn.
    p.; cm.
  Includes bibliographical references and index.
  ISBN 978-0-470-67424-6 (pbk.)
I. Quinn, Joseph F., 1962–, editor of compilation.   II. Title.
[DNLM: 1. Dementia. WM 220]
  RC521
  616.8′3–dc23
                                                    2013019917

A catalogue record for this book is available from the British Library.

Wiley also publishes its books in a variety of electronic formats. Some content that appears in print may not be available in electronic books.

Cover image: © iStockphoto.com/Eraxion
Cover design by Sarah Dickinson Design

Set in 8.75/11.75pt Utopia by SPi Publisher Services, Pondicherry, India
Printed and bound in Malaysia by Vivar Printing Sdn Bhd

1   2014

Contents

Contributors

Anahita Adeli, MD
Department of Neurology
Mayo Clinic
Rochester, MN, USA

Ira Byock, MD
Dartmouth-Hitchcock Medical Center
Lebanon, NH, USA

Richard Camicioli, MD, FRCPC
Department of Neurology
University of Alberta
Edmonton, Alberta, Canada

Elizabeth Crocco, MD
Departments of Neurology and Psychiatry
and Behavioral Sciences,
Miller School of Medicine, University of Miami,
Miami, FL, USA

Ranjan Duara, MD
Wien Center for Alzheimer's Disease and Memory
Disorders, Mount Sinai
Medical Center; Departments of Neurology and
Psychiatry and Behavioral Sciences, Miller School
of Medicine, University of Miami;
Department of Neurology, Herbert Wertheim
College of Medicine, Florida International
University
Miami, FL, USA

Linda Ganzini, MD, MPH
Portland Veterans Affairs Medical Center,
Oregon Health and Science University
Portland, OR, USA

Cory Ingram, MD, MS
Mayo Clinic, College of Medicine
Mankato, MN, USA

Keith A. Josephs, MD, MST, MSc
Department of Neurology
Mayo Clinic, College of Medicine
Rochester, MN, USA

Jason Karlawish, MD
Departments of Medicine and Medical Ethics,
Perelman School of Medicine at the University
of Pennsylvania
Philadelphia, PA, USA

Anne M. Lipton, MD, PhD
Diplomate in Neurology, American Board of
Psychiatry and Neurology
Vancouver, British Columbia, Canada

David A. Loewenstein, PhD
Wien Center for Alzheimer's Disease and
Memory Disorders, Mount Sinai Medical Center;
Departments of Neurology and
Psychiatry and Behavioral Sciences,
Miller School of Medicine,
University of Miami
Miami, FL, USA

Joel Mack, MD
Department of Psychiatry, Oregon Health
and Science University
Portland, OR, USA

David Mansoor, MD
Portland Veterans Affairs Medical Center, Oregon
Health and Science University
Portland, OR, USA

Andrew McKeon, MD
Department of Laboratory Medicine and Pathology
Mayo Clinic, College of Medicine
Rochester, MN, USA

Sahana Misra, MD
Portland Veterans Affairs Medical Center, Oregon
Health and Science University
Portland, OR, USA

Amie Peterson, MD
Department of Neurology, Oregon Health
and Science University
Portland, OR, USA

Amy May Lin Quek, MD
Department of Laboratory Medicine and Pathology
Mayo Clinic, College of Medicine
Rochester, MN, USA

Joseph Quinn, MD
Department of Neurology, Oregon Health and
Science University
Portland, OR, USA

Murray A. Raskind, MD
Department of Psychiatry and Behavioral Sciences,
University of Washington
Seattle, WA, USA

Norman Relkin, MD, PhD
Department of Neurology and Neuroscience
Weill Medical College of Cornell University
New York, NY , USA

Amy Y. Tsou, MD
Department of Neurology, Perelman School of
Medicine at the University of Pennsylvania
Philadelphia, PA, USA

Daniel Varon, MD
Wien Center for Alzheimer's Disease and Memory
Disorders, Mount Sinai Medical Center;
Department of Neurology, Herbert Wertheim
College of Medicine, Florida International
University
Miami, FL, USA

Lucy Y. Wang, MD
Department of Psychiatry and Behavioral Sciences,
University of Washington
Seattle, WA, USA

Clinton Wright, MD
Departments of Neurology and Psychiatry and
Behavioral Sciences, Miller School of Medicine,
University of Miami,
Miami, FL, USA

Series Foreword

The genesis for this book series started with the proposition that, increasingly, physicians want direct, useful information to help them in clinical care. Textbooks, while comprehensive, are useful primarily as detailed reference works but pose challenges for uses at the point of care. By contrast, more outline-type references often leave out the "hows and whys" – pathophysiology, pharmacology – that form the basis of management decisions. Our goal for this series is to present books, covering most areas of neurology, that provide enough background information to allow the reader to feel comfortable, but not so much as to be overwhelming; and to associate that with practical advice from experts about care, combining the growing evidence base with best practices.

Our series will encompass various aspects of neurology, with topics and the specific content chosen to be accessible and useful.

Chapters cover critical information that will inform the reader of the disease processes and mechanisms as a prelude to treatment planning. Algorithms and guidelines are presented, when appropriate. "Tips and Tricks" boxes provide expert suggestions, while other boxes present cautions and warnings to avoid pitfalls. Finally, we provide "Science Revisited" sections that review the most important and relevant science background material, and references and further reading sections that guide the reader to additional material.

We welcome feedback. As additional volumes are added to the series, we hope to refine the content and format so that our readers will be best served.

Our thanks, appreciation, and respect go out to our editors and their contributors, who conceived and refined the content for each volume, assuring a high-quality, practical approach to neurological conditions and their treatment.

Our thanks also go to our mentors and students (past, present, and future), who have challenged and delighted us; to our book editors and their contributors, who were willing to take on additional work for an educational goal; and to our publisher, Martin Sugden, for his ideas and support, for wonderful discussions and commiseration over baseball and soccer teams that might not quite have lived up to expectations. We would like to dedicate the series to Marsha, Jake and Dan; and to Janet, Laura and David. And also to Steven R. Schwid, MD, our friend and colleague, whose ideas helped to shape this project and whose humor brightened our lives, but he could not complete this goal with us.

Robert A. Gross
Jonathan W. Mink
Rochester, NY, USA

Preface

This book is the culmination of an effort to meet the request for a brief, practical clinician's guide to dementia. As in clinical practice, we start with "Diagnosis," the traditional responsibility of the neurologist. Chapter 1 is an overview reiterating practice parameters and standard guidelines, but we recognize that the cases that cause practicing neurologists to reach for a textbook are the atypical ones. After considering the categories of atypical cases most often referred to memory disorder clinics, we devoted the next several chapters to the special problems of dementias with rapid progression, young onset, features suggestive of normal pressure hydrocephalus, the pseudodementia of depression, and prodromal dementia or MCI. Throughout these first six chapters there is an emphasis on the treatable possibilities, with the goal of helping clinicians to recognize these important (if rare) cases.

While the neurologist's role in dementia is often confined to the diagnosis, Chapter 7 explicitly describes the potential role of the neurologist in the continuing care of dementia patients. This overview is followed by more detailed discussions of the use of psychotropic drugs and palliative care, relying on our colleagues from psychiatry and palliative care to cover two practical topics which are not addressed in most neurology textbooks. These chapters are intended to provide tips for medical management of dementia patients, but as practicing clinicians appreciate, the management of dementia goes beyond medicine, with legal and ethical considerations presenting a number of non-"medical" challenges for clinicians to navigate, so Chapter 10 is devoted to this important topic.

The last two chapters look to the future of dementia care and in some ways are "works in progress." Chapter 11 reviews options for monitoring outcomes in dementia, a likely necessity for clinical practice as health care systems move toward an emphasis on patient outcomes for reimbursement. The final chapter addresses the issue of dementia prevention, providing something of a roadmap for clinicians to provide to the worried children of adult patients who either serve as caregivers or who show up in clinic asking for early assessment and intervention.

We selected these chapter topics based on the questions most often referred to us in a memory disorders clinic from practicing neurologists. The goal was not to be comprehensive but to be helpful to clinicians. During the initial planning phases of the book, some reviewers voiced concerns that it would be outdated before it was printed, as disease-modifying therapy would be approved by now and completely change the landscape of dementia care. We sincerely hope that this text does become obsolete as clinical research advances, but in the meantime trust that these efforts will assist practicing clinicians with the challenge of caring for patients with dementia.

Diagnosis and Differential Diagnosis of Dementia

Richard Camicioli

Department of Medicine (Neurology), University of Alberta, Canada

Introduction

The burden of dementia, a substantial public health concern, is felt in all societies. After defining dementia, in the following chapter we discuss the diagnosis and differential diagnosis. We outline an approach to the general diagnostic work-up in this chapter, with detailed recommendations for specific situations (e.g. rapid progression, young onset, prominent depression, question of normal pressure hydrocephalus) in the chapters to follow.

Definitions

Dementia is a syndrome in which multiple-domain cognitive impairment, generally including memory impairment, is sufficiently severe to significantly affect everyday function. Memory and one additional area of cognitive impairment, including aphasia, apraxia, agnosia, and executive dysfunction, are required to be affected according to common criteria (DSM-IV). There are other generic dementia criteria, including the ICD-10 criteria,which require that several domains are affected, and newer dementia criteria are being developed (i.e. DSM-V) (Table 1.1). Some criteria have not required memory impairment as a necessary condition for dementia, since it might not be prominently impaired in non-Alzheimer's dementias, and even occasional patients with Alzheimer's disease can exceptionally have relatively preserved memory.

There are specific criteria for patients with cerebrovascular disease (vascular cognitive impairment/ vascular dementia) and Parkinson's disease (Parkinson's disease dementia - PDD), both of which have a high risk of dementia. Recently, new criteria for Alzheimer's disease (AD) have been proposed to take into account developments in biomarkers and recognition of a prodomal state, termed mild cognitive impairment, which often leads to dementia. Dementia with Lewy bodies (DLB) shares pathologies of Parkinson's disease and Alzheimer's disease. Frontotemporal dementia also has distinct features and varied pathology, and typically presents with prominent behavioral features (behavioral variant frontotemporal dementia) or language impairment (non-fluent/agrammatic/ logopenic primary progressive aphasia or semantic dementia). Some patients, particularly those with logopenic progressive aphasia, actually have Alzheimer's disease pathology. Some frontotemporal dementia patients develop co-existent motor neuron disease. Progressive supranuclear palsy (PSP), corticobasal ganglionic degeneration (CBGD), and Huntington's disease are other neurodegenerative disorders that usually have obvious and prominent motor features; patients with these conditions often have cognitive and behavioral problems and develop dementia. Thus, while diagnostic criteria for the dementias are in evolution, making a diagnosis and identifying the specific etiology remain critical in the clinical setting.

Distinct pathologies can be successfully identified by current clinical criteria, albeit with a rate of misdiagnosis. The recognition of unusual presentations, atypical onset, and the prodromal phase of dementias may be assisted by biomarkers (which may differ in these settings). Clinicians must

Dementia, First Edition. Edited by Joseph F. Quinn.
© 2014 John Wiley & Sons, Ltd. Published 2014 by John Wiley & Sons, Ltd.

Table 1.1 Comparison of key guidelines for the assessment of dementia

Guideline	Mental status	Activities of daily living	Behavioral symptoms	Blood tests	Brain imaging	Other tests
AAN, 2001	Yes	No specific recommendation	Depression screen	CBC, TSH, B12, glucose, electrolytes, BUN/Cr, liver function tests	Structural imaging	Selective
Canadian Consensus, 2004	Yes	No specific recommendation, but highlights dementia is a clinical diagnosis	No specific recommendation, but highlights dementia is a clinical diagnosis	B12, TSH, electrolytes, calcium, glucose	CT or MRI: <60, rapid onset (<2 mo), short duration (<2yrs), head trauma, neurological signs or symptoms, urinary incontinence, gait disorder, cancer, anticoagulants, atypical cognitive features	Selective
European Federation of Neurology, 2010	Yes, and assess specific domains	Yes	Yes	B12, folate, TSH, calcium, glucose, CBC, renal and liver tests	CT or MRI may be used	Dopamine SPECT scan to differentiate AD and LBD

AD, Alzheimer's disease; BUN, blood urea nitrogen; CBC, complete blood count; CR, creatine; CT, computed tomography; LBD, Lewy body dementia; MRI, magnetic resonance imaging; SPECT, single photon emission computed tomography; TSH, thyroid-stimulating hormone.

nevertheless recognize these possibilities. Also, it is important to keep in mind that overlapping pathology often occurs in older patients with cognitive impairment or dementia, which might influence the clinical picture.

Other chapters consider young-onset and rapidly progressive dementia. Here we consider dementia in people 65 years of age and older.

⚙ SCIENCE REVISITED

The clinical diagnosis of Alzheimer's diease is confirmed at brain autopsy in 90% of patients. The clinical diagnosis of vascular dementia, Lewy body dementia, and frontotemporal dementia predicts the brain autopsy diagnosis, but not as well as a clinical diagnosis of Alzheimer's.

Epidemiology

In 2010, dementia was estimated to affect 35.7 million people world-wide. Alzheimer's disease is the most common dementia in people older than age 65 years, yet Alzheimer's disease pathology is often accompanied by vascular disease or Lewy bodies. The latter two types of dementia can also occur in "pure" form. The diagnosis of dementia increases mortality risk, regardless of age or etiology of dementia. It is important to recognize that dementia may lead to a debilitated state and death in order to direct interventions appropriately, including palliative approaches. Prediction of death can be challenging in patients with dementia, which may make initiation of formal palliative care services difficult. (Chapter 9 provides a detailed discussion of the role of palliative care in dementia.)

Assessment

History

Obtaining an accurate medical history is central to the diagnosis of dementia. This should identify and qualify the nature of the symptoms as well as their onset and progression. A critical challenge to obtaining an accurate history is that patients themselves may not be able to self-monitor because of their cognitive problems, so obtaining a collateral history is necessary. Memory impairment is a central feature of many dementias and can be

expected to interfere with recall of key historical events. In addition, lack of insight can occur in dementia and interfere with the acknowledgment of symptoms. It is important to interview the informant and patient separately at some point in the diagnostic process. While some standardized questionnaires are useful in identifying complaints, these do not replace a thorough history, which remains the gold standard. Instruments that can complement the clinical history include the AD8 dementia screening questionnaire, the Informant Questionnaire on Cognitive Decline in the Elderly (IQCODE), the Deterioration Cognitive Observation Scale (DECO), and the Alzheimer Questionnaire (AQ). The General Practitioner Assessment of Cognition (GPCog) includes both a cognitive screen and questions regarding cognitive changes and activities of daily living based on caregiver report, which improves sensitivity and specificity for the diagnosis of dementia.

While the initial focus of the history should be on cognitive complaints and their functional implications, which allow for meeting dementia criteria, psychiatric and behavioral changes need to be identified as they are often present in early dementia, and can be prominent in some patients. In many patients referred for cognitive decline, psychiatric issues may predominate and may be the cause of the so-called cognitive decline. Depression should routinely be assessed in patients with cognitive complaints. It is key to screen for depressive symptoms, and scales such as the Geriatric Depression Scale, which has 15- and 30-item versions (www.stanford.edu/~yesavage/GDS.html), and the Montgomery-Asberg Depression Scale, can be helpful in this regard, though the gold standard is a psychiatric evaluation using a standardized interview schedule. The Cornell Scale for Depression in Dementia is validated for the dementia population. Depression can be a risk factor for or coincident with the diagnosis of dementia. Moreover, it can occur *de novo* in the course of dementia. Although they are distinct symptoms, depression and anxiety often co-exist. Other mood symptoms, such as elation or euphoria, also can occur in dementia, but primary psychiatric disorders should be kept in the differential diagnosis if these are prominent.

While not absolute, the nature of cognitive deficits can help in differentiating depression from dementia. Patients with depression have long response latencies whereas typical patients with Alzheimer's disease respond with normal latencies. Memory impairment in depression is related to retrieval problems, rather than problems with encoding, where cueing does not improve recall. Alzheimer's patients also have additional cognitive deficits, particularly in visuospatial and language domains, that would not be seen in depression. As noted, depression can co-exist with dementia and it is common in Alzheimer's disease as well as vascular dementia and dementia with Lewy bodies.

Other neuropsychiatric problems that should be considered include positive symptoms such as disinhibition, irritability, agitation, aggression, or abnormal motor behavior as well as negative symptoms such as apathy. Delusions and hallucinations are also highly relevant. These symptoms can be assessed using standardized instruments such as the Neuropsychiatric Inventory (NPI). They can occur early in the course of dementia and can evolve over time. The Frontal Behavior Inventory can help with the differentiation of Alzheimer's disease from frontotemporal dementia. Patients with frontotemporal dementia often lack emotional responsiveness and can develop apathy, which can be mistaken for depression but is characterized by lack of motivation. Psychotic features, particularly visual hallucinations, are characteristic of PDD and DLB. Delusions are not as specific but can be equally disturbing to family members.

It is critical to identify functional impairment. By definition, patients with mild cognitive impairment (MCI) do not have substantial functional impairment, while patients with dementia do. Practically speaking, at the time of diagnostic evaluation, assessment of basic and instrumental activities of daily living is performed by asking the patient and their caregiver how the patient performs everyday tasks. Basic activities of daily living such as getting in and out of bed, dressing, walking, toileting, bathing, and eating are not affected early in the course of dementia. Instrumental activities of daily living (IADL) such as answering the phone, taking pills, handling money, shopping, cooking, and driving are affected early in the course.

Typically a standardized questionnaire is used to address activities of daily living. Examples include the Functional Activities Questionnaire (FAQ) which addresses IADLs, the Lawton and Brody IADL and Physical Self-Maintenance Scale and the OARS Functional Assessment Questionnaire. Assessment is not as straightforward as it seems, as there is often a mild degree of functional impairment in MCI, where such impairments may predict future cognitive decline. Moreover, a given patient's living situation might not tax their functional capacity. Conversely, a patient who is working might have some workplace impairment despite relatively well-preserved cognitive assessment. In the setting of a disorder that affects motor function, such as Parkinson's disease or after a stroke, it can be challenging to determine if a change in a patient's function is related to cognitive or motor function.

Prescribed and over-the-counter medications, as well as substances of abuse (notably alcohol), are important to identify as they might contribute to cognitive impairment. If the patient is not able to list these accurately, this suggests an important area of functional impairment that requires intervention. All co-morbid medical conditions need to be identified. Vascular risk factors such as smoking, diabetes, obesity, hyperlipidemia, hypertension, atrial fibrillation, and non-central nervous system (CNS) vascular disease (cardiac, renal, peripheral) increase the risk for cerebrovascular events, which can contribute to dementia, and can be covert. These are risk factors for dementia in the absence of identifiable stroke as well. Symptoms suggestive of cancer, especially in patients with a rapid course, raise the concern of direct or indirect central nervous system involvement.

A detailed family history is critical. While familial dementia commonly has a young onset, risk of dementia in older people is also increased in the setting of a family history. A third to half of people with frontotemporal dementia have a family history compared to roughly one in 10 patients with Alzheimer's disease. At a minimum, all first-degree relatives should be identified and the presence of neurological disorders determined. This history should not be restricted to examining dementia risk, since disorders such as Parkinson's disease and motor neuron disease may be associated with an increased risk of dementia in family members. If the family history is consistent with a hereditary dementia, testing can be offered but this should be done after appropriated counseling. At-risk family members should only be tested after genetic counseling. Huntington's disease is a relatively common cause of dementia in younger individuals, but can occasionally be identified for the first time in older patients without an obvious family history.

Physical examination

General examination

The general examination might identify specific co-morbid conditions, such as atrial fibrillation, congestive heart failure or chronic obstructive pulmonary disease (COPD). An abdominal or rectal mass, suggesting a neoplasm, might be uncovered. These might directly or indirectly contribute to cognitive dysfunction. Some findings on general examinations, such as postural hypotension, may suggest a specific diagnosis such as dementia with Lewy bodies.

Cognitive evaluation

Cognitive assessment at the bedside is important for both differential diagnosis and rating the severity of cognitive impairment. Cognitive domains to be assessed correspond to those involved in the diagnosis, including attention, orientation, memory, executive function, language, praxis, and visuospatial abilities.

Several standardized assessment instruments have improved clinicians' abilities to assess cognition. While these are helpful, the clinician needs to be able go beyond such instruments at times, given their limitations in scope and sensitivity. The Mini-Mental Status Examination (MMSE) is the most commonly used instrument and its advantages include its widespread use and extensive validation. Disadvantages include its relative insensitivity to the diagnosis of dementia, which may be partly related to exclusion of some cognitive domains, such as executive function. Given the availability of superior instruments, its use will likely decrease over time. The MMSE may not be sensitive to memory impairment since it only relies on the immediate recall of three words. Expanded versions of the MMSE such as the 3MS might have increased sensitivity. More comprehensive standardized instruments include the Short Portable Mental Status Examination, the Montreal Cognitive Assessment (MOCA) (www.mocatest.org), and the Addenbrooke Cognitive Examination-Revised. The Frontal Assessment Battery evaluates aspects of frontal lobe function, and can be used as a complement to tools such as the MMSE that do not specifically address this cognitive domain. It can assist in the differentiation of AD from frontotemporal dementia and may be useful in assessing parkinsonian disorders.

Neuropsychological testing, which affords a comprehensive, objective, and standardized approach to quantifying cognitive impairment, is helpful for diagnosis and differential diagnosis, but is not available in all settings. It is particularly relevant in mild or questionable cases, in cases where malingering is suspected, or in subjects for whom ceiling or floor effects might obscure interpretation of results on simplified tests (for example, people with very high or very low levels of education). Patients with clear changes and obvious deficits on simpler tests may not require neuropsychological testing. Moreover, it should be borne in mind that subjects may have test scores that are abnormal based on statistical population-based comparison but that this may represent a "normal" score or minimal change for that individual. Neuropsychological tests can be helpful in following change over time. The shorter tests do not necessarily validly assess cognitive subdomains as can be done by neuropsychological batteries, which may be important in differential diagnosis.

> ### ✭ TIPS AND TRICKS
>
> When should neuropsychological tests be used?
>
> - In patients with worrisome history but good performance on mental status exam.
> - In cases where malingering is suspected.
> - To distinguish depression with cognitive symptoms from neurodegenerative disease.

Neurological examination

A complete general neurological examination is important. On cranial nerve testing, olfactory deficits are common in Lewy body dementia. Visual field defects or higher order visual defects may suggest cerebrovascular disease affecting the visual pathways or a posterior evolving dementia, such as the visual variant of AD or the Heidenhain variant of Creutzfeldt–Jakob disease (CJD). Other cranial nerve examination clues to the etiology of dementia can include vertical supranuclear gaze difficulty suggesting progressive supranuclear palsy. Nystagmus and restricted eye movement can be seen in Wernicke's encephalopathy, which can evolve into alcoholic dementia. Gaze-evoked nystagmus is non-specific and be seen with many causes of cerebellar degeneration. Upper motor neuron facial weakness suggests pyramidal involvement. Lower motor neuron facial weakness and involvement of other lower cranial nerves may provide a clue to involvement of the subarachnoid space due to an inflammatory, neoplastic or infectious process. Bulbar difficulties are seen in processes involving the brainstem or upper motor neuron lesions.

Focal weakness with other pyramidal signs can be seen in patients with cerebrovascular disease. Pyramidal signs can also be a clue to the presence of motor neuron disease (amyotrophic lateral sclerosis – ALS), in which features of lower motor neuron dysfunction can also be found (fasciculations, atrophy). Up to 10% of frontotemporal dementia patients can develop features of ALS, which has a substantial impact on prognosis and hence on long-term planning.

Cerebellar dysfunction in dementia might indicate a specific neurodegenerative disorder such as multiple system atrophy, a paraneoplastic disorder, CJD or celiac disease.

Neuropathy can be seen in renal failure, diabetes, vitamin B12 deficiency, alcohol exposure or paraneoplastic disorders. Neuropathy can also be seen in HIV, Lyme disease or hepatitis C infections which all can be associated with cognitive impairment and dementia. In addition, some mitochondrial disorders or disorders of central white matter (leukodystrophies) can be associated with neuropathy. Mitochondrial disorders are also classically associated with myopathy, myoclonus, and seizures.

Gait assessment is critical in patients with dementia. While it is less often impaired in AD, it is commonly affected in PDD, vascular dementia, and dementia with Lewy bodies.

It is important to examine for adventitious movements. The triad of tremor (rest tremor), bradykinesia, and rigidity indicates parkinsonism, as seen in dementia with Lewy bodies or Parkinson's disease. Chorea would suggest Huntington's disease, neuroacanthocytosis or another Huntington-like disorder. Dystonia in older adults may suggest a cerebrovascular event, either in the basal ganglia or thalamus. In addition to dystonia, unilateral chorea or tremor in an older adult should lead to consideration of a cerebrovascular event or other lesion, generally involving frontostriatal circuits, which can additionally be involved in cognition.

Myoclonus can be seen in degenerative disorders, including advanced AD and DLB, and more rarely Huntington's disease and frontotemporal dementia. Focal myoclonus as well as asymmetrical apraxia, parkinsonism, and dystonia is characteristic of corticobasal ganglionic degeneration. Myoclonus is included in the diagnostic criteria of CJD, though it may not be seen early in the illness. When CJD is considered, it is important to keep alternative entities in mind. In terms of systemic illness, myoclonus is most often a manifestation of any cause of encephalopathy, including common disorders such as renal or hepatic disease (asterixis), as well as rarer autoimmune disorders such as steroid-responsive encephalopathies associated with thyroid disease or antibodies to the CNS. Rare disorders such as mitochondrial disease are characterized by myoclonus.

Laboratory studies

Blood and spinal fluid

Recommended tests for the assessment of dementia include blood work-up, including complete blood count (CBC), glucose, electrolytes (including calcium), renal and hepatic tests and thyroid function. Testing for vitamin B12 or folate deficiency is recommended. In many areas grains are supplemented with folate, making folate deficiency unlikely unless there are other reasons for malabsorption, in which case malabsorption of other B-vitamins should be considered. If indicated, based on the patient's history, assessment for chronic infections that can cause dementia, such as HIV or syphilis, is indicated.

If the presentation suggests a delirium additional testing should be done to rule out possible causes of delirium such as acute infections (cultures, chest x-ray, urinalysis). Work-up for inflammatory or autoimmune disorders should also be considered. The erythrocyte sedimentation rate (ESR), C-reactive protein (CRP) or more specific tests such as rheumatoid factors and antinuclear antibodies can provide clues to the presence of an autoimmune disorder. Additional work-up is indicated if specific disorders such as vasculitis, Sjögren's syndrome, sarcoidosis or a paraneoplastic or non-paraneoplastic autoimmune encephalopathies are being considered.

A complete work-up may include cerebrospinal fluid (CSF) examination, which can also be used to seek evidence for acute or subacute infections, autoimmune or inflammatory disorders or neoplastic involvement of the central nervous system. While proteins in the CSF, such as beta-amyloid, tau and phosphorylated tau, can be used to provide evidence for AD, these tests are not currently used routinely. This may change as additional evidence accumulates for their utility in treatment decisions, and they become more readily available. The use of CSF markers in the differential diagnosis of CJD is controversial, because the markers (14-3-3, tau, S100B) are non-specific. Nevertheless, CSF examination is important in rapidly progressive dementia to rule out or rule in treatable dementia and the CSF markers may improve diagnostic certainty in the appropriate clinical context.

Imaging

Structural imaging (computed tomography [CT] or magnetic resonance imaging [MRI]) scans can rule out structural contributions to cognitive decline (stroke, subdural hematoma, tumors) and are increasingly being used to "rule in" specific diagnoses, when atrophic or vascular changes are observed that are consistent with a particular dementia diagnosis. While MRI is more sensitive than CT, CT scans can still provide meaningful information. For example, vascular changes, subdural hematomas and many tumors, while better delineated on MRI, can be seen quite well on modern CT scans. Similarly hydrocephalus can be identified on CT in cases of suspected normal pressure hydrocephalus (NPH). In NPH and other forms of hydrocephalus, MRI allows examination of the posterior fossa to search for lesions that might lead to obstruction of CSF flow. An absence of ventricular enlargement on CT can exclude NPH and help to redirect further investigation and diagnostic considerations. A caution in interpreting ventricular enlargement is that it might be due to global atrophy.

In addition to better resolution, specific MRI approaches (such as gradient echo MRI) can identify findings such as cerebral microbleeds, which are not evident on CT. These suggest amyloid angiopathy and are often seen in association with white matter disease, which is found patients with vascular cognitive impairment or dementia. MRI imaging might help to discern an atrophy pattern consistent with degenerative syndromes such as progressive supranuclear palsy PSP,

multiple system atrophy (MSA) or corticobasal ganglionic degeneration. Brain atrophy is less prominent in DLB and PDD than in AD and it is not prominent in PD until cognitive decline ensues. On the other hand, atrophy is prominent in frontotemporal lobar degenerations.

Dopamine transporter imaging (^{123}I-fluoropropyl-2-beta-carbomethoxy-3-beta(4-iodophenyl)nortropane single photon emission computed tomography: FP-CIT SPECT) is useful in differentiating DLB from dementias that do not affect the dopaminergic system. Functional studies examining perfusion (Tc-hexamethylpropyleneamine oxime [HMPAO] SPECT) or glucose metabolism (fluorodeoxyglucose [FDG] positron emission tomography [PET]) provide additional information that can be useful in the differential diagnosis of dementia. Building on previous work with the C-11 compound Pittsburgh Compound B (PIB), the availability of readily accessible ligands, such as F-18-fluorbetapir, that can bind amyloid will likely assist in differential diagnosis but, as with all imaging modalities, will have to be interpreted in the clinical context. Newer techniques are becoming available that examine brain networks and their connectivity.

Types of dementia

Specific features of the history, examination, and investigations can assist in the differential diagnosis of dementia (Figure 1.1, Table 1.2). After reversible conditions have been ruled out, the clinician should attempt to make a specific diagnosis of dementia type. The most common causes of dementia are Alzheimer's disease, vascular dementia, Lewy body dementia, and frontotemporal dementia. Here some features of particular importance are discussed.

✋ CAUTION

Be vigilant about the possibility of treatable diagnoses, even though these are quite rare with dementia. Other chapters include more detailed discussion of treatable entities like depression and NPH, or treatable encephalopathies presenting as rapidly progressive dementia or young-onset dementia.

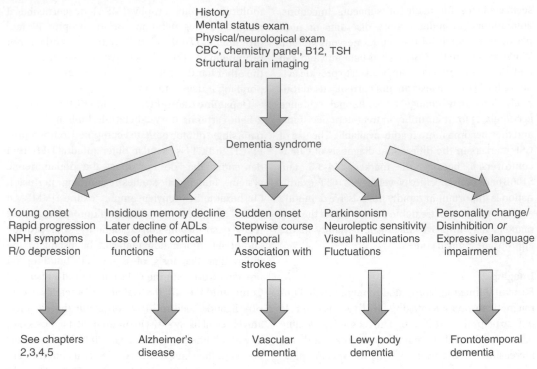

Figure 1.1 General approach to differential diagnosis of dementia.

Alzheimer's disease

Alzheimer's disease typically presents with insidiously progressive memory impairment, which eventually involves executive function and visuospatial function. Involvement of memory and at least one other cognitive domain is necessary. In addition, the cognitive deficits must be sufficient to affect function, distinguishing it from mild cognitive impairment. A key is that there should be no other specific cause of the cognitive impairment, such as a delirium or a psychiatric disorder, a principle that holds for all primary degenerative dementias. The AD criteria have been revised recently given the realization that pathological changes likely precede clinically manifest disease by years, if not decades. In addition, the new revision acknowledges that behavioral changes, in additional to cognitive changes, may interfere with function. Among developments since the 1984 criteria were published is refinement of the diagnosis of frontotemporal lobar degeneration and dementia with Lewy bodies, which now have their own criteria. It is acknowledged that rare patients might meet criteria for a specific dementia diagnosis and yet have positive biomarkers for a different one.

While AD is most commonly a memory disorder, focal cortical presentations are common, especially in younger patients. The differential diagnosis of this group of patients may be aided by biomarkers that can be used to indicate Alzheimer pathology, with the caveat that mixed pathology would not be excluded.

Some patterns are highly suggestive of Alzheimer pathology, while others suggest alternative pathology. Posterior cortical atrophy is associated with prominent visual impairment with visual agnosia and Balint syndrome (asimulagnosia, visual ataxia, and ocular apraxia) and is commonly associated with AD, though DLB pathology may also lead to impaired visuospatial function. The Heidenhain variant of CJD is also characterized by visuospatial impairment.

Vascular dementia

Vascular dementia is diagnosed when the presence of strokes is confirmed and when the clinician judges that the vascular events are responsible for

Table 1.2 Selected features allowing differential diagnosis of dementia

	Alzheimer's disease	Frontotemporal dementia	Dementia with Lewy bodies	Vascular dementia	Creutzfeldt–Jakob disease
Cognitive features	Memory predominates	Behavior and executive function and language	Relative sparing of memory, with executive and visuospatial	Localization dependent, but executive dysfunction predominates	Rapidly progressive cognitive and motor impairment
Memory impairment	+++	+	+	+/-	+/-
Executive dysfunction	+	+++	++	++	+/-
Visuospatial impairment	+	–	+++	+/-	++
Neurological signs	Absent early, may occur later	In those with motor neuron disease	Present in majority	Typically present	Defining criterion
Pyramidal	–	+ With motor neuron disease	–	+++	++
Extrapyramidal	+	+ In familial frontotemporal lobar degeneration	+++ Defining criterion	+	++
Cerebellar signs	–	–	–	+/-	++
Lower motor neuron signs	–	+	–	–	+/-

cognitive decline. The prototype of vascular dementia has an acute onset and stepwise decline, with focal neurological signs and symptoms, but this entity is rarely seen in clinical practice. It is important to note that vascular risk factors or atherosclerosis are not sufficient for a diagnosis of vascular dementia; the brain parenchyma has to be damaged by infarcts in order for this diagnosis to be appropriately applied. Diffuse white matter changes (leukoaraiosis) can also lead to vascular cognitive impairment, often gradually progressive and associated with mood changes, gait impairment and urinary frequency or incontinence.

Lewy body dementia

Lewy body dementia is distinguished by the presence of parkinsonism, neuroleptic sensitivity, fluctuations in consciousness, and spontaneous (i.e. not drug induced) visual hallucinations, although patients vary in the specific combinations of signs and symptoms. In contrast to idiopathic Parkinson's disease, the parkinsonism in Lewy body dementia tends to occur in the absence of rest tremor, is more symmetrical, and does not respond as well to dopaminergic drugs. The diagnosis of Lewy body dementia is also reserved for patients whose motor symptoms have been present for less than 1 year when dementia appears, in contrast to the 8–10 years of motor symptoms without dementia in idiopathic PD, which typically precedes PDD. Other features suggestive of Lewy body dementia include disproportionate visuospatial dysfunction and rapid eye movement (REM) behavior disorder.

Frontotemporal dementia

Frontotemporal dementia may present as either a language impairment or a behavioral variant. Progressive aphasia due to frontotemporal pathology is characterized by either progressive non-fluent speech (progressive non-fluent aphasia) or loss of knowledge of the meaning of items (semantic dementia). They typically have a young onset, and can develop behavioral features and asymmetrical focal atrophy, which suggest frontotemporal dementia but these features are insensitive. Criteria for possible behavioral variant frontotemporal dementia (bvFTD) include combinations of prominent behavioral features such as disinhibition, apathy or inertia, loss of sympathy or empathy, perseveration or compulsions, hyperorality or executive dysfunction. Relative sparing of episodic memory and visuospatial function are cognitive features of bvFTD. It should be kept in mind, however, that hippocampal pathology, distinct from AD, can be found in bvFTD. Supportive features include functional impairment sufficient to indicate dementia (which allows differentiation from primary psychiatric disorders), and imaging showing frontal or anterior temporal atrophy or hypometabolism in a pattern consistent with the diagnosis increases the likelihood of probable bvFTD.

Problems with current classifications

The current diagnostic criteria are not absolute in terms of specificity or sensitivity (see Table 1.1). Some scenarios may suggest an acute CNS disorder, yet be due to a degenerative dementia. Abrupt onset suggests delirium, which needs to be ruled out to make a diagnosis of dementia; however, delirium may be a precursor to dementia and is more common in the setting of dementia. Abrupt decline can occur in DLB, where fluctuating cognition may lead to a marked deterioration. In some, this might be precipitated by an acute infection or medications, which can lead to diagnostic confusion. Delirium increases the risk of mortality in older people. Cerebrovascular disease also can present acutely, and can lead to cognitive decline. A difficulty with the diagnosis of vascular dementia is establishing a temporal association between cerebrovascular disease and dementia, given that vascular events can be undetected without imaging in some patients, despite their contribution to cognitive decline.

A patient with incipient dementia of any kind is susceptible to delirium. In such patients, a prolonged recovery, possible to a lower level of cognitive function, may occur. While a typical patient with AD has a decline of three points on the MMSE annually, more rapid progression can be seen. When present, like acute onset, this should prompt a search for potentially treatable entities. Rapidly progressive dementias are discussed in detail in Chapter 2. Co-morbid conditions are also a reality in older populations and may influence the course of dementia but also compromise a confident diagnosis. Nevertheless, a progressive course despite medical illness should not preclude the diagnosis of degenerative dementia. Similar concerns apply in psychiatric illness, in which a late-life degenerative dementia can occur.

Focal presentations can also lead to diagnostic confusion and uncertainty. Presentation with focal symptoms is characteristic of frontotemporal dementia and corticobasal ganglionic degeneration. Focal presentations can also occur in AD, in which language impairment, characterized by paucity of speech (which needs to be differentiated from primary progressive aphasia), apraxia (which needs to be differentiated from corticobasal ganglionic degeneration) and visuospatial impairment, which is common in DLB, are not uncommon. Overlapping pathologies, including AD, vascular changes and Lewy bodies, present in a large proportion of patients with dementia, and can confound the clinical picture.

Biomarkers

While biomarkers have been available for decades, evidence is accumulating that they can be useful in the differential diagnosis of dementia. Currently most biomarkers require further validation in order to be applied clinically beyond the research setting. Beyond causal genes that are associated with autosomal dominant disease (APP, PSEN1, PSEN2), genetic risk factors exist for AD and likely for other dementias as well. Possession of an apolipoprotein E4 (APOE 4) allele is a well-established risk factor in AD. Recently identified risk alleles include alterations in complement component (3b/4b) receptor-1 (CR1), clusterin (CLU) and phosphatidylinositol binding clathrin assembly protein (PICALM), each of which may provide a hint regarding pathophysiology. For example, they may point to inflammation, lipid metabolism or trafficking of organelles. Other polymorphisms are being identified but while these may be important scientifically, they are not helpful in the clinic at present.

Blood markers are less strongly associated with the development of dementia. Since the blood–brain barrier impedes transmission of markers between the brain and blood, it is not surprising that these markers may not be as sensitive as spinal fluid markers. Nevertheless, they may be helpful in identifying potential risk factors, if not patterns related to disease. Levels of plasma amyloid, particularly beta-amyloid fragments 1-42 and 1-40, or their ratio, have been inconsistently associated with increased risk of dementia. Other markers include those for oxidative stress, inflammation, glucose metabolism, lipid metabolism, B-vitamin metabolism (i.e. homocysteine), etc. In frontotemporal dementia, low progranulin levels are found in some patients, in whom they can predict the presence of mutations. Developments in large-scale proteomic and metabolomic screening will likely identify marker patterns associated with specific dementias. These may be applicable to blood or cerebrospinal fluid but currently these approaches are not clinically available.

Cerebrospinal fluid is adjacent to the brain and might be expected to better reflect CNS pathology. As noted above, CSF examination is indicated if an inflammatory, neoplastic or infectious etiology is suspected in the evaluation of a patient. If NPH is suspected, large-volume CSF drainage may help diagnostically. CSF markers can be helpful in differentiating AD from other forms of dementia such as frontotemporal dementia or Lewy body dementia, albeit with overlap. Specifically, low CSF amyloid (1-42) concentrations are suggestive of Alzheimer pathology. Increases in total tau (t-tau) and phosphorylated-tau (p-tau) are also present in AD but these intraneuronal proteins can also reflect neuronal damage and are therefore elevated in any pathological processes that destroy brain tissue.

Current research is examining forms of beta-amyloid and tau as prognostic markers in cognitively normal individuals and people with mild cognitive impairment. Additional markers have been examined and are likely to be developed. As with the blood markers, these may provide insights into distinct pathologies and pathophysiological processes.

Imaging

As noted above, structural brain imaging is an important part of the initial evaluation of patients with suspected dementia. Assistance in differential diagnosis and use as a marker in tracking disease are also potential goals of brain imaging. MRI can identify hippocampal atrophy which correlates with the presence of AD pathology. Overall, the challenge with use of biomarkers is their relative timing in relation to clinical disease. For example, some changes, like amyloid deposition, might occur presymptomatically with little change through the disease course, whereas others, such as global brain atrophy, might be evident only after the disease is in place. These concepts apply across dementias with different markers or diagnostic signatures at play.

While positron emission tomography (PET) is not routinely used, fluorodeoxyglucose (FDG) PET scans can assist in differential diagnosis as can technetium-HMPAO SPECT, which measures cerebral blood flow. These approaches are particularly helpful in differentiating AD, which shows posterior hypoperfusion or decreased metabolism, from frontotemporal dementia, which shows frontal changes, and vascular dementia, which shows patchy changes. Dementia with Lewy bodies is more challenging to differentiate, likely because of overlapping AD pathology in many cases. Nevertheless, the pattern of change in Lewy body dementia may be distinct, with occipital hypometabolism or decreased blood flow. In addition to assisting in the differentiation of different types of dementia, metabolic imaging may be helpful in identifying patients with early cognitive decline at risk for transitioning to dementia of the Alzheimer type. The recent advent of practical ligands that allow imaging of amyloid using PET will likely assist in identifying patients with pathological changes of AD.

Parkinsonian disorders, related to loss of striatal dopamine function, can be separated from other dementing disorders such as AD. Currently dopamine transporter imaging using SPECT or PET imaging dopamine metabolism using 18-F-dopa or presynaptic dopamine transporter using 11-C-dihydrotetrabenazine (DHTBZ) are helpful, but have been most widely used in the research setting. Readily available dopamine transporter imaging with SPECT has lead to more widespread use despite the caveat that such changes might not separate different parkinsonian disorders. Cardiac imaging using metaiodobenzylguanidine (MIBG) shows loss of uptake in Lewy body-related disorders but, like blood flow (HMPAO) and dopamine transporter imaging using SPECT, this method might not offer adequate sensitivity or specificity on its own.

Future of dementia diagnosis

The diagnosis of dementia is a clinical decision. The increased availability of imaging and other modalities will likely prove helpful, but they will not supplant clinical decision making based on key aspects of the history and physical examination.

Further reading

Carcaillon L, Berrut G, Sellal F, et al. Diagnosis of Alzheimer's disease patients with rapid cognitive decline in clinical practice: interest of the DECO questionnaire. *J Nutr Health Aging* 2011; **15**(5): 361–6.

Clark CM, Schneider JA, Bedell BJ, et al, for the AV45-A07 Study Group. Use of florbetapir-PET for imaging beta-amyloid pathology. *JAMA* 2011; **305**(3): 275–83.

Cummings JL, Mega M, Gray K, Rosenberg-Thompson S, Carusi DA, Gornbein J. The Neuropsychiatric Inventory: comprehensive assessment of psychopathology in dementia. *Neurology* 1994; **44**(12): 2308–14.

Dubois B, Burn D, Goetz CG, et al. Diagnostic procedures for Parkinson's disease dementia: recommendations from the Movement Disorder Society Task Force. *Mov Disord* 2007; **22**: 2314–24.

Dubois B, Slachevsky A, Litvan I, Pillon B. The FAB: a Frontal Assessment Battery at bedside. *Neurology* 2000; **55**(11): 1621–6.

Feldman HH, Jacova C, Robillard A, et al. Diagnosis and treatment of dementia: 2. Diagnosis. *Can Med Assoc J* 2008; **178**(7): 825–36.

Galvin JE, Roe CM, Powlishta KK, et al. The AD8: a brief informant interview to detect dementia. *Neurology* 2005; **65**(4): 559–64.

Goldman JS, Hahn SE, Catania JW, et al, for the American College of Medical Genetics and the National Society of Genetic Counselors. Genetic counseling and testing for Alzheimer disease: joint practice guidelines of the American College of Medical Genetics and the National Society of Genetic Counselors. *Genet Med* 2011; **13**(6): 597–605.

Hort J, O'Brien JT, Gainotti G, Pirttila T, et al, for the EFNS Scientist Panel on Dementia. EFNS guidelines for the diagnosis and management of Alzheimer's disease. *Eur J Neurol* 2010; **17**(10): 1236–48.

Jack CR, Knopman DS, Jagust WJ, et al. Hypothetical model of dynamic biomarkers of the Alzheimers pathological cascade. *Lancet Neurol* 2010; **9**(1): 119–28.

Jack CR Jr, Albert MS, Knopman DS, et al. Introduction to the recommendations from the National Institute on Aging-Alzheimer's Association workgroups on diagnostic guidelines for Alzheimer's disease. *Alzheimers Dement* 2011; **7**(3): 257–62.

Kertesz A, Davidson W, Fox H. Frontal behavioral inventory: diagnostic criteria for frontal lobe dementia. *Can J Neurol Sci* 1997; **24**(1): 29–36.

Knapskog AB, Barca ML, Engedal K. A comparison of the validity of the Cornell Scale and the MADRS in detecting depression among memory clinic patients. *Dement Geriatr Cogn Disord* 2011; **32**(4): 287–94.

McKeith IG, Dickson DW, Lowe J, et al, for the Consortium on DLB. Diagnosis and management of dementia with Lewy bodies: third report of the DLB Consortium. *Neurology* 2005; **65**(12): 1863–72.

McKhann GM, Knopman DS, Chertkow H, et al. The diagnosis of dementia due to Alzheimer's disease: recommendations from the National Institute on Aging-Alzheimer's Association workgroups on diagnostic guidelines for Alzheimer's disease. *Alzheimers Dement* 2011; 7(3): 263–9.

Rascovsky K, Hodges JR, Knopman D, et al. Sensitivity of revised diagnostic criteria for the behavioural variant of frontotemporal dementia. *Brain* 2011; **134**(Pt 9): 2456–77.

Román GC, Tatemichi TK, Erkinjuntti T, et al. Vascular dementia: diagnostic criteria for research studies. Report of the NINDS-AIREN International Workshop. *Neurology* 1993; **43**(2): 250–60.

Sabbagh MN, Malek-Ahmadi M, Kataria R, et al. The Alzheimer's questionnaire: a proof of concept study for a new informant-based dementia assessment. *J Alzheimers Dis* 2010; **22**(3): 1015–21.

Sikkes SA, van den Berg MT, Knol DL, et al. How useful is the IQCODE for discriminating between Alzheimer's disease, mild cognitive impairment and subjective memory complaints? *Dement Geriatr Cogn Disord* 2010; **30**(5): 411–16.

Teng EL, Chui HC. A Modified Mini-Mental State (3MS) Examination. *J Clin Psychiatry* 1987; **48**: 314–18.

2

Rapidly Progressive Dementia and its Mimics

Amy May Lin Quek and Andrew McKeon

Department of Laboratory Medicine and Pathology, Mayo Clinic College of Medicine, USA

Introduction

An expedited and comprehensive evaluation of a patient with rapid loss of cognitive function is critical to determining whether or not they have a treatable disorder. In this chapter, we will explore the differential diagnosis of rapidly progressive dementia (RPD, Figure 2.1); clinical features and clues helpful in the diagnostic process; and therapies initiated for potentially reversible disorders. A recent review of over 1000 brain autopsy cases referred to the US National Prion Disease Pathology Surveillance Center (at Case Western Reserve) demonstrated a treatable cause for dementia in 7% of cases. Most common among those treatable disorders were immune-mediated diseases including autoimmune encephalitis and primary angiitis of the central nervous system (CNS), followed by neoplasia and CNS infection. Much of the progress in recent years pertaining to early identification of reversible forms of RPD has emerged because of availability of anti-body biomarkers aiding an autoimmune diagnosis. Frequently these diagnoses are missed, treatments are not initiated in a timely manner, and duration of treatment is too short. Thus there is an emphasis on evaluation and management of autoimmune dementias herein.

Definitions

Dementia refers to a disorder characterized by cognitive and/or behavioral impairment significantly affecting activities of daily living. Etiologies are diverse, and thus the term dementia is not exclusive to neurodegenerative causes. Definitions of RPD vary in case series of patients studied or in review articles by experts in the field, but most authors seem to include patients who reach severe dementia or death no later than 18 months to 4 years after symptom onset. In clinical practice, patients with RPD present with subacute onset of cognitive or behavioral symptoms, with significant disability accruing week by week.

Epidemiology

Precise data regarding frequency of RPDs are not available, but these disorders seem uncommon in comparison to slowly progressive dementias. In 6 years, 178 patients with RPD were evaluated in a specialized center (University California San Francisco [UCSF]). Over a 10-year period, 22 patients aged 17–45 years with RPD were evaluated at the Mayo Clinic. At the same institution, 22 patients with a neurodegenerative RPD were evaluated over an 8-year period. Among the UCSF cohort, sporadic Creutzfeldt–Jakob disease (CJD) accounted for the majority of patients evaluated (47%), other neurodegenerative etiologies were second most common (15%), and autoimmune diseases third (8.4%). Among non-prion neurodegenerative RPDs, frontotemporal lobar degeneration (FTLD, with or without motor neuron degeneration), progressive supranuclear palsy (PSP), corticobasal degeneration (CBD), diffuse Lewy body disease (DLBD), and Alzheimer's disease (AD) were all demonstrated pathologically at autopsy. In the Case Western

Dementia, First Edition. Edited by Joseph F. Quinn.

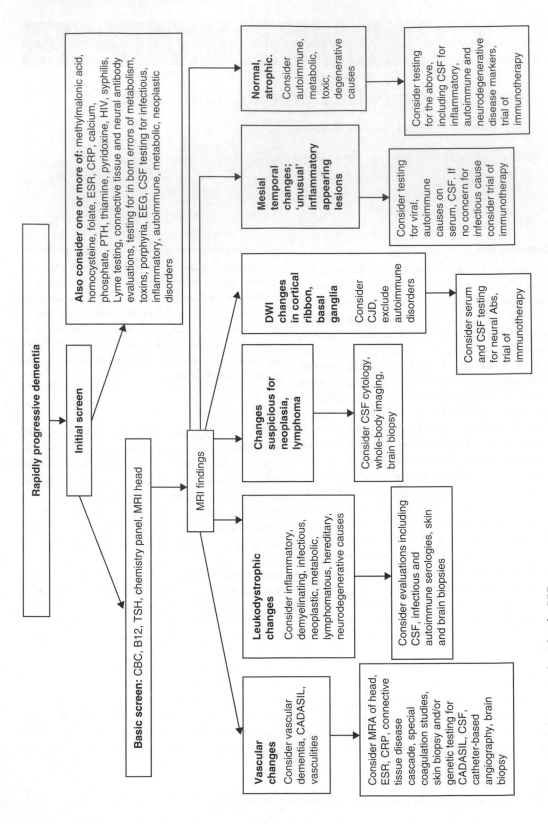

Figure 2.1 A diagnostic algorithm for RPD.

Rapidly progressive dementia

Initial screen

Basic screen: CBC, B12, TSH, chemistry panel, MRI head

Also consider one or more of: methylmalonic acid, homocysteine, folate, ESR, CRP, calcium, phosphate, PTH, thiamine, pyridoxine, HIV, syphilis, Lyme testing, connective tissue and neural antibody evaluations, testing for in born errors of metabolism, toxins, porphyria, EEG, CSF testing for infectious, inflammatory, autoimmune, metabolic, neoplastic disorders

MRI findings

Vascular changes
Consider vascular dementia, CADASIL, vasculitis

Consider MRA of head, ESR, CRP, connective tissue disease cascade, special coagulation studies, skin biopsy and/or genetic testing for CADASIL, CSF, catheter-based angiography, brain biopsy

Leukodystrophic changes
Consider inflammatory, demyelinating, infectious, neoplastic, metabolic, lymphomatous, hereditary, neurodegenerative causes

Consider evaluations including CSF, infectious and autoimmune serologies, skin and brain biopsies

Changes suspicious for neoplasia, lymphoma

Consider CSF cytology, whole-body imaging, brain biopsy

DWI changes in cortical ribbon, basal ganglia
Consider CJD, exclude autoimmune disorders

Consider serum and CSF testing for neural Abs, trial of immunotherapy

Mesial temporal changes; 'unusual' inflammatory appearing lesions

Consider testing for viral, autoimmune causes on serum, CSF. If no concern for infectious cause consider trial of immunotherapy

Normal, atrophic.
Consider autoimmune, metabolic, toxic, degenerative causes

Consider testing for the above, including CSF for inflammatory, autoimmune and neurodegenerative disease markers, trial of immunotherapy

Reserve autopsy series, AD (14%) and vascular dementia (3%) were the most common neuropathological diagnoses after prion disease, while treatable disorders collectively accounted for 6.4% of patients. Detected diseases, in order of commonality, were immune-mediated disorders, neoplasia, infections, and metabolic disorders. Thirty-five percent of patients with immunotherapy-responsive autoimmune dementia are initially diagnosed as having neurodegenerative or prion disorders prior to recognition.

> ✋ CAUTION
>
> Rapidly progressive dementia does not mean CJD. The premature diagnosis of CJD is to be avoided. Recent pathological studies have demonstrated that 7% of patients who come to autopsy with a clinical diagnosis of CJD had a treatable cause. A list of treatable causes (Figure 2.1) needs to be carefully considered and excluded. Cerebrospinal fluid (CSF) 14,3,3 protein is a non-specific marker of neuronal damage and reliance on this as the sole evidence for a CJD diagnosis is hazardous.

Spongiform disorders

Creutzfeldt–Jakob disease is a rapidly progressive prion disorder of the CNS. Most patients have a sporadic form, although cases may be hereditary (5–15% of cases), iatrogenic (rare, occurring by transmission from infected corneal transplants, pooled cadaveric pituitary hormones, dural grafts, and electroencephalogram depth electrodes), and transmitted from cows infected with bovine spongiform encephalopathy (variant-CJD; younger onset-age [20s], and frequent psychiatric and sensory symptoms early on). For the sporadic form, average onset-age is 65 years, and sexes are affected equally. Clinical presentations vary, but the most frequent are changes in behavior and cognition, often followed by abnormalities in vision. Dementia and muteness usually ensue quickly, and myoclonus is prominent. Cerebellar ataxia (Oppenheimer variant) or visuospatial difficulties (Heidenhain variant) may predominate initially. The diagnosis rests on typical clinical findings, magnetic resonance imaging (MRI) abnormalities, and the exclusion of alternative causes. Routine CSF tests

are normal; the diagnostic utility of 14-3-3 protein, S100B, and neuron-specific enolase (NSE) testing on CSF is controversial, with concerns regarding specificity of these tests. Data from the Case Western Reserve autopsy cohort suggest that 50% of patients with a potentially treatable disorder, previously diagnosed as CJD, had an elevated 14-3-3 protein.

Electroencephalogram (EEG) findings include an evolving pattern of diffuse slowing to high-voltage triphasic sharp wave (usually 1–2 Hz) complexes, that give the appearance of periodicity (pseudoperiodic). The latter EEG findings, though characteristic, typically appear during late stages of the disease.

Recent data suggest that cortical ribbon and deep lenticular nuclear diffusion-weighted (most striking) and fluid-attenuated inversion recovery (FLAIR) imaging abnormalities are the most sensitive and specific findings for CJD.

Rare spongiform disorders include Gerstmann–Straussler–Scheinker syndrome (autosomal dominant inheritance, chronic course with prominent corticospinal tract and extrapyramidal signs and relatively mild dementia) and fatal familial insomnia (autosomal dominant inheritance, rapid course with intractable insomnia and dementia).

Other rapidly progressive neurodegenerative dementias

At autopsy of patients with RPD, pathological evidence of neurodegenerative disorders other than prion disease is frequently detected. At the UCSF RPD unit, neurodegenerative disease (non-prion related) was responsible for 14.6% of all patients referred for suspected CJD and represented 39% of the non-prion cases. The Mayo Clinic series of 22 patients diagnosed with RPD showed that 23% of the cases consisted of frontotemporal dementia with motor neuron disease, 18% had either CBD or PSP, 14% had DLBD, and 9% had AD. In the Case Western Reserve autopsy cohort, AD accounted for over half of patients with a rapidly progressive incurable dementia diagnosed in life as CJD; other diagnoses in the non-prion neurodegenerative group were (in order of commonality) neurodegenerative disorder not otherwise specified, FTLD, DLBD, tauopathy not otherwise specified, PSP, CBD, and Huntington's disease (HD).

Diagnostic clues useful for neurodegenerative disorders such as AD, DLBD, PSP, and CBD are usually unreliable when the clinical course is rapidly progressive. Illness duration beyond 12 months may be indicative of a neurodegenerative disorder other than CJD. In one series of six patients with RPD and autopsy diagnosis of DLBD, half presented with acute confusion to an emergency room. In the Mayo Clinic RPD series, patients with DLBD were distinguishable from other neurodegenerative causes on the basis of a transient postoperative or illness-related encephalopathy having occurred 2 years prior to the dementia onset. In the same series, parkinsonism, psychosis, rapidly fluctuating cognition (all typical of DLBD), and motor neuron disease (classically encountered in FTLD) were seen in patients with AD and CJD, and myoclonus was observed exclusively in CJD patients. Contrary to this, another series of autopsy-proven rapidly progressive DLBD demonstrated that half had myoclonus.

Indeed, multifocal signs, motor signs, psychosis, apathy, apraxia, and seizures have all been reported as signs predicting rapid progression in patients with AD in general. Other factors that have been reported to be associated with a rapidly progressive course in AD (all controversial) include co-morbid cardiovascular disease, diabetes mellitus, high educational level, low educational level, and severe cognitive impairment at disease onset. CSF measures associated with rapid cognitive decline in AD include high total tau or phosphorylated tau, low beta-amyloid Abeta1-42, and a high ratio of total tau to Abeta1-42.

Atypical presentations of other heredodegenerative disorders

Carriers of premutations of the FMR1 gene typically present with ataxia and intention tremor (the fragile X-associated tremor/ataxia syndrome). A syndrome dominated by RPD (executive dysfunction, apathetic behavior in addition to mild ataxia) has been described in two patients.

Psychiatric and cognitive changes may be initial manifestations of HD preceding motor signs by many years. The clinical presentation to a neurologist may be that of personality change, mood disturbance, and altered work performance. Although usually indolent in onset, physical or psychological stress may lead to fairly acute unmasking of clinical symptoms or signs. One patient with a RPD accompanied by generalized myoclonus, generalized tonic-clonic seizures, and ataxia was reported to have Unverricht–Lundborg disease, a form of progressive myoclonic epilepsy.

Autoimmune causes of rapidly progressive dementia

Autoimmune diseases may involve cerebral structures crucial for memory, cognition, and behavior. Careful consideration of autoimmune disorders presenting as RPD is important, since they are potentially amenable to immunotherapy if treated early.

Clinical terminology varies and includes autoimmune encephalitis, autoimmune dementia, limbic encephalitis (LE), paraneoplastic encephalopathy, and steroid-responsive encephalopathy with autoimmune thyroiditis (SREAT, aka Hashimoto encephalopathy). Over the last decade, identification of novel neural autoantibodies targeting proteins involved in synaptic transmission and plasticity has led to heightened awareness of autoimmune causes of cognitive impairment. Since many neural autoantibodies have only been identified recently, the phenotypical range of their associated neurological disorders continues to broaden.

In one series, young-onset dementia was attributed to autoimmune and inflammatory causes in 20% of patients. All ages can be affected; the largest study of voltage-gated potassium channel complex (VGKC) antibody seropositive patients reported a median onset-age of 65 years. Clinical presentations are heterogeneous and frequently multifocal.

Clinical manifestations

Patients with autoimmune neurological disorders may present acutely or subacutely. LE, a well-recognized autoimmune neurological disorder, is characterized by subacute short-term memory loss, neuropsychiatric disturbances (irritability, depression, hallucinations, personality change), and temporal lobe seizures.

In cases atypical for LE, an autoimmune cause may be overlooked. Other cognitive domains that may be affected in autoimmune encephalitis include learning, abstract reasoning, executive function, gnosis, and praxis. Attention deficits and impaired consciousness (delirium) are also commonly encountered in autoimmune cognitive decline, but their absence should not preclude the diagnosis of an autoimmune neurological disorder. The course of autoimmune dementia may fluctuate.

As accompanying neurological and psychiatric features are often encountered, history of behavioral changes, psychiatric symptoms (such as hallucination and mood changes), insomnia, movement disorders, seizures, and neuropathy should be obtained. In some, the multifocal neurological involvement may emerge only with temporal progression of the autoimmune disease. Personal or family history of autoimmunity and cancer are risk factors for autoimmune dementia, and their presence is helpful to raise further suspicion of an autoimmune etiology.

The clinical evaluation of cognitive function, using a cognitive test such as the Mini-Mental State Exam (MMSE) or Kokmen Short Test of Mental Status, should demonstrate impairments in one or more domains of cognition. Brainstem signs, myoclonus, ataxia, myelopathy, and peripheral somatic and autonomic neuropathy may be present. These features, indicative of a multifocal neurological involvement, may further trigger consideration of autoimmunity. A thorough clinical evaluation to search for non-neurological autoimmunity (alopecia, thyroid disease, vitiligo, systemic lupus erythematosus) should be performed.

Etiology and pathogenesis

When detected, neural-specific autoantibodies may serve as markers of the immune-mediated process. Neurological involvement may also be seen in non-organ specific autoimmune disorders, such as systemic lupus erythematosus and Sjogren syndrome; neural autoantibodies may not be detected in this setting.

Neural autoantibodies associated with autoimmune dementias

Neural autoantibodies (Plate 2.1) may be broadly classified under two categories, based on the location of antigenic targets: antibodies that target intracellular antigens (Table 2.1) and antibodies that target neural cell surface proteins or receptors (Table 2.2).

SCIENCE REVISITED

Neural antibodies that target intracellular antigens are not pathogenic, as the intracellular target antigens are inaccessible to the circulating antibodies during life. Rather, these antibodies are markers of a T cell-predominant immune response mediated by

CD8+ cytotoxic T cells. The presence of these antibodies often suggests a paraneoplastic process, they may co-exist with other neural autoantibodies, and the antibody profile predicts the cancer type. Removal of a detected cancer generally stops or slow disease progression, but reversal of the neurological deterioration is rare, even when immunotherapy is administered. Commonly detected antibodies in this category are antineuronal autoantibody type 1 (ANNA-1), Ma/Ta antibodies (Ma1 and Ma2, or Ma2 alone), and collapsin-response mediator-protein 5-(CRMP5)-IgG.

SCIENCE REVISITED

In contrast to antibodies that target intracellular antigens, antibodies directed at cell surface antigens may alter the structure or function of the corresponding neural antigens, and play direct pathogenic roles in mediating the neurological disorders, including cognitive impairment and dementia (see Table 2.2). The diagnostic work-up of a patient who presents with rapidly progressive dementia should include testing for these antibodies, as many of them target antigens that are receptors or their associated protein complexes involved in synaptic transmission and plasticity. Neurological disorders mediated by these autoantibodies are often reversible and amenable to antibody-depleting therapies. Many of these neural autoantibodies were recently identified and their associated range of neurological disorders continues to expand.

VGKC antibodies

Early associations of VGKC autoantibodies included peripheral nerve hyperexcitability (Isaacs syndrome, acquired neuromyotonia), Morvan syndrome, and LE. The cancer association of VGKC antibodies is relatively low in frequency (20–30%) and diverse in the range of tumors seen.

Cognitive impairment is the most common neurological manifestation, and these patients may present with a syndrome of RPD. Cognitive and neuropsychiatric manifestations include executive

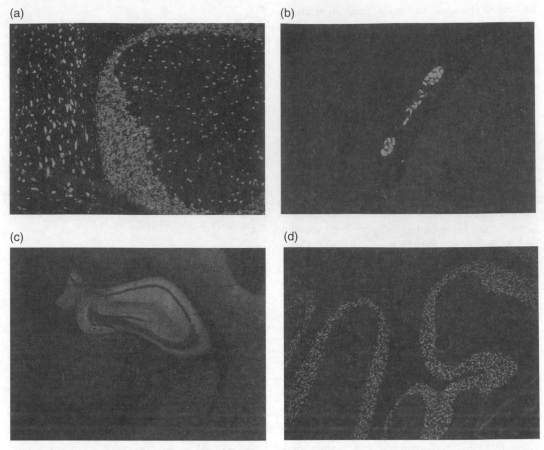

Plate 2.1 Distribution of autoantibody immunoreactivity for ANNA-1 and NMDA receptor antibody in mouse neural tissues. ANNA-1 binds primarily to neuronal nuclei of cerebellar Purkinje, granular layer and molecular layer neurons (a, *right*), midbrain neurons (a, *left*) and myenteric plexus neurons (b). NMDA receptor antibody binds to neural synapses primarily in hippocampus (c) and cerebellar granular layer (d). (*see insert for color representation of the plate.*)

dysfunction, disorientation, agnosia, memory impairment, behavioral and personality changes (irritability, apathy, lethargy, aggression), depression, anxiety, hallucinations, and impaired attention. Seizures may be temporal or extratemporal in origin. Other multifocal neurological manifestations may occur. A hallmark feature described in these patients is the syndrome of inappropriate antidiuretic hormone secretion (SIADH) that is secondary to hypothalamic involvement.

Given the diverse multifocal neurological accompaniments of patients with VGKC autoantibodies, patients who present with RPD frequently resemble neurodegenerative disorders, including frontotemporal dementia-like syndrome and CJD. Even when the clinical syndrome fulfills the diagnostic criteria

for CJD, including cortical diffusion-weighted imaging hyperintensities, VGKC autoimmunity should be ruled out.

Recently, it was reported that target antigens in many patients with VGKC antibodies are proteins structurally and functionally associated with the channel. These antibodies target leucine-rich, glioma-inactivated 1 (Lgi1) and contactin-associated protein 2 (Caspr2) proteins. Clinical manifestations reported in association with Lgi1-IgG are LE (including presentation with RPD mimicking CJD), myoclonus, faciobrachial dystonic seizures, epilepsy, and hyponatremia. Caspr2-IgG has been described in patients with encephalitis, peripheral nerve hyperexcitability or both. Patients with encephalitis have been described to have subacute

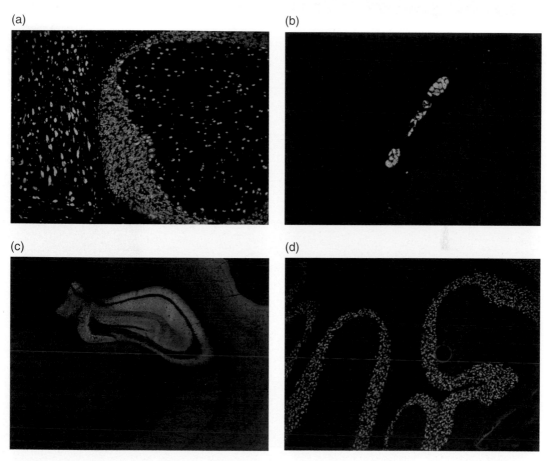

Plate 2.1 Distribution of autoantibody immunoreactivity for ANNA-1 and NMDA receptor antibody in mouse neural tissues. ANNA-1 binds primarily to neuronal nuclei of cerebellar Purkinje, granular layer and molecular layer neurons (a, *right*), midbrain neurons (a, *left*) and myenteric plexus neurons (b). NMDA receptor antibody binds to neural synapses primarily in hippocampus (c) and cerebellar granular layer (d).

Dementia, First Edition. Edited by Joseph F. Quinn.
© 2014 John Wiley & Sons, Ltd. Published 2014 by John Wiley & Sons, Ltd.

Table 2.1 Neural autoantibodies targeting intracellular antigens reported to present with cognitive impairment, accompanying neurological findings and oncological associations

Antibody	Cognitive disorders	Other neurological manifestations	Cancer association
ANNA-1 (Hu)	Limbic encephalitis (LE)	Peripheral neuropathy (most commonly sensory), cerebellar syndrome; cranial neuropathy	Small cell carcinoma; thymoma Neuroblastoma (children)
ANNA-2 (Ri)	Dementia LE Encephalopathy	Brainstem encephalitis, cerebellar disorder, myelopathy, peripheral neuropathy	Breast adenocarcinoma, small cell carcinoma
ANNA-3	LE	Peripheral neuropathy (sensory/ sensorimotor), cerebellar ataxia, brainstem encephalitis, myelopathy	Small cell carcinoma, adenocarcinoma (lung or esophagus)
PCA-1 (Yo)	Cognitive impairment, personality change (rare)	Cerebellar disorder, brainstem encephalitis, cranial neuropathy, peripheral neuropathy	Müllerian carcinoma, breast carcinoma
PCA-2	LE	Brainstem encephalitis, cerebellar disorder, Lambert–Eaton syndrome, peripheral and autonomic neuropathies	Small cell carcinoma
Amphiphysin	Cognitive dysfunction, encephalopathy, LE	Neuropathy, myelopathy, stiff-person phenomena, Lambert–Eaton syndrome	Small cell lung carcinoma, breast adenocarcinoma
CRMP-5	Subacute dementia, personality change	Seizures, chorea, ataxia, psychiatric, cranial neuropathy (optic neuropathy, abnormal olfaction/taste), myelopathy, radiculopathy, neuropathy, Lambert–Eaton syndrome	Small cell carcinoma, thymoma
Ma1, Ma2	Memory impairment, dementia, LE	Brainstem encephalitis, cerebellar syndrome, hypothalamic disorder, psychiatric symptoms	Testicular germ cell tumors (MA2); lung, gastrointestinal, non-Hodgkin lymphoma, breast (MA1)
GAD65	LE	Seizures, cerebellar ataxia, brainstem, stiff-person phenomena, extrapyramidal signs, myelopathy	*Thymoma, renal cell, adenocarcinoma (breast or colon)
AGNA (SOX1)	LE	Lambert–Eaton syndrome, cerebellar dysfunction	Small cell lung carcinoma

*GAD65 antibody syndromes are more commonly idiopathic, although paraneoplastic cases have been reported.

Table 2.2 Neural autoantibodies targeting cell membrane antigens reported to present with cognitive impairment, accompanying neurological findings and oncological associations

Antibody	Cognitive disorders	Other neurological manifestations	Cancer association
VGKC antibody (antigenic targets may be Lgi1, CASPR2)	Limbic encephalitis (LE), amnesia, executive dysfunction Dementia (including frontotemporal dementia-like syndrome and Creutzfeldt–Jakob-like disease)	Seizures, psychiatric, insomnia, extrapyramidal disorder, myoclonus, hypothalamic disorder, autonomic disorders, peripheral hyperexcitability	Small cell lung cancer, thymoma, prostate, adenocarcinoma, breast adenocarcinoma
NMDA receptor antibody	Memory impairment Psychosis Agitation	Characteristic multistage syndrome of prodrome, psychiatric symptoms, seizures, abnormal movements (including orofacial dyskinesia), followed by decreased responsiveness, hypoventilation and autonomic instability	Ovarian teratoma
GABA$_B$ receptor antibody	Memory impairment, behavioral problems (LE)	Seizures (LE), visual hallucinations, aphasia, orolingual movements, cerebellar ataxia	Small cell lung carcinoma Neuroendocrine neoplasia
AMPA receptor antibody	Memory loss, disorientation, behavioral change, agitation (LE)	Seizures (LE), nystagmus, hypersomnia, progressive unresponsiveness, dysdiadochokinesia, hallucinations	Breast, lung, thymus
mGlur5	LE	Seizures	Lymphoma
Ganglionic acetylcholine receptor antibody	Cognitive impairment, executive dysfunction, frontotemporal syndrome, encephalopathy	Dysautonomia, peripheral neuropathy	Adenocarcinoma, renal cell carcinoma, lymphoid cancers

progressive memory difficulties, personality changes, and seizures.

NMDA receptor antibody encephalitis

Autoantibodies to the N-methyl D-aspartate receptor (NMDAR) were first identified in 12 women with memory and psychiatric disturbances, decreased consciousness, and ovarian teratoma in 2007. NMDAR-IgG targets the NR1 (GluN1) subunit of the NMDAR, an ionotropic glutamate-gated cation channel that plays an important role in synaptic plasticity and excitotoxicity, mediating cognition, behavior, motor, respiratory, and autonomic control. This disorder is probably one of the most frequent among the neurological autoimmune encephalopathies.

Patients who develop rapidly progressive cognitive deterioration in NMDAR antibody encephalitis

(NMDARAE) usually have a distinctive constellation and symptom evolution. Typically, the illness begins with prodromal symptoms, comprising fever, headache, upper respiratory and gastrointestinal symptoms, before patients develop psychiatric symptoms and memory impairment. One or more of seizures, abnormal movements (especially orofacial dyskinesias), autonomic instability, hypoventilation, and coma may follow.

While the distribution of patients with NMDARAE is highest in the young adult age groups, children and the elderly may also be affected. Female sex, 20s–40s age group, and African American race are risk factors for the detection of tumor, typically ovarian teratoma. Seventy-five percent of patients recover from this severe illness with immunotherapy and tumor removal (if present), although the recovery process is protracted and neurological dysfunction may persist, especially if treatment is delayed. Up to 25% of patients relapse, and risk for relapse increases in patients with no prior immunotherapy at onset, undetected tumor or rapid immunotherapy taper.

Diagnostic approach

In a patient with suspected autoimmune RPD, the diagnostic work-up is directed to finding objective evidence to support this diagnosis (clinically, radiologically, and on serum or CSF) and cancer detection. Parallel work-up to rule out other causes of rapidly progressive cognitive decline, especially those that are reversible, should also be performed. Brain imaging, EEG, and neuropsychometric testing can also provide baseline, objective parameters that can be followed over time as the patient receives treatment, to help evaluate treatment efficacy.

Autoantibody testing

Comprehensive neural autoantibody testing should be performed on serum and CSF. Selective isolated antibody testing is not advised, as the range of autoantibodies associated with acute cognitive decline is diverse and autoantibodies may co-exist. The neural antibody profile facilitates the identification of a paraneoplastic etiology (see Tables 2.1 and 2.2). An important caveat is that non-detection of a neural antibody does not exclude the diagnosis of autoimmune encephalitis when other clinical clues are evident.

> ### ★ TIPS AND TRICKS
>
> Neural autoantibodies should be tested on serum, CSF or both. Certain antibodies, such as NMDA receptor antibodies, are more readily detected on CSF. When suspicion is high and serological tests are negative, consideration should be given to CSF screening for neural autoantibodies in order to increase the diagnostic yield.

Testing for non-neural autoantibodies should also be performed. Detection of non-neural autoantibodies may support an autoimmune diagnosis, although the antibodies are unlikely to be directly relevant from a neuropathophysiological standpoint. For example, in patients with SREAT, thyroperoxidase (TPO) antibodies may be the only ones identified. A marker for an autoimmune condition, these antibodies do not directly cause the encephalopathy but their detection should prompt consideration for a trial of immunotherapy. Furthermore, detection of non-neural antibodies may facilitate the diagnosis of a non-organ specific autoimmune process with neuropsychiatric manifestations, such as systemic lupus erythematosus, but other clinical features to support the diagnosis should be elicited.

Neuroimaging

Magnetic resonance imaging typically demonstrates T2/ FLAIR hyperintensities involving the medial temporal lobes in LE (Figure 2.2a), but extratemporal involvement may also occur. Mild gadolinium enhancement of the affected areas may be detected; meningeal enhancement has been reported in patients with NMDARAE. Subsequent MRIs performed to follow up the signal changes may demonstrate lesion resolution or resultant atrophy. When the medial temporal region is affected, serial MRIs may develop radiographic changes that are indistinguishable from hippocampal sclerosis.

In some patients, the MRI remains normal or demonstrates only minimal changes despite the severity of their symptoms. Serial MRIs may sometimes demonstrate radiological changes that lag behind the clinical presentation. Functional imaging, such as positron emission tomography (PET) and single photon emission computed tomography (SPECT), may demonstrate regions of abnormal brain metabolism.

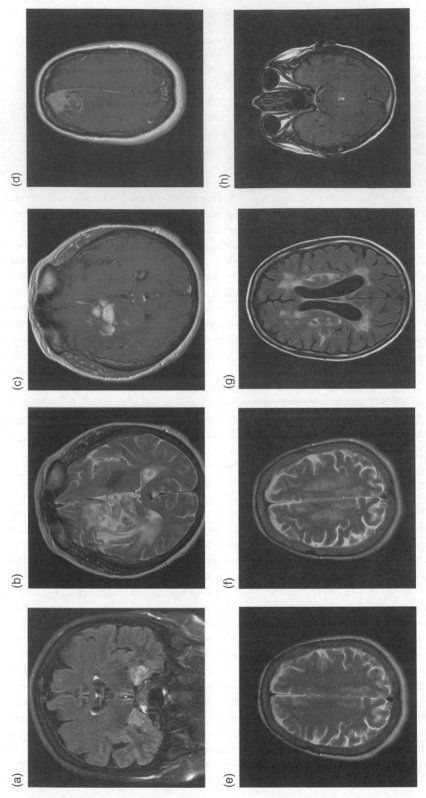

Figure 2.2 MRI images of FIVE patients with RPD. (a) Coronal T2 FLAIR demonstrates high signal in bilateral hippocampi in a patient with LE. (b) (T2 axial) and (c) (T1 postgadolinium axial) images demonstrate a patient with primary CNS lymphoma. (d) T1 postgadolinium axial image of a patient with a highly vascular and rapidly growing right frontal meningioma. MRI T2 axial pre (e) and 12 months post (f) whole-brain irradiation for small cell carcinoma. T2 FLAIR images demonstrating diffuse signal abnormalities of white matter (g) in a patient with CADASIL, including the anterior temporal lobes (h).

Electrophysiology

The eletroencephalogram (EEG) is not specific for an autoimmune diagnosis, as the changes are non-specific and may comprise focal or generalized slowing and interictal epileptiform discharges. Similar to the MRI findings, these changes may originate from both temporal and extratemporal regions. A clinically important use of the EEG is to differentiate encephalopathy from non-convulsive or subtle seizures in patients whose symptoms are fluctuating and episodic. The EEG should be reviewed carefully for electrographic seizures, and in some cases, prolonged video-EEG monitoring may be indicated.

Cerebrospinal fluid measures

Cerebrospinal fluid evaluation may add further information supportive of an autoimmune process. Abnormalities that may be found include elevated protein concentration (the range can reach >100 mg/dL), elevated white cell count (usually lymphocyte predominant), CSF-exclusive oligoclonal bands, elevated IgG index and synthesis. These are non-specific findings seen in many neurological inflammatory disorders but, when present, would be supportive of an autoimmune neurological disorder.

Cancer screening

Factors that predict the type and likelihood of tumor detection are the antibody profile (see Tables 2.1 and 2.2), and the patient's sex, age, and risk factors (in particular smoking history). Screening with CT of the thorax, abdomen and pelvis, mammogram for women, and testicular ultrasound for men are recommended. If these are negative in the presence of a paraneoplastic autoantibody, further screening with PET-CT scan may be considered as this increases diagnostic yield of a cancer by 20%. Other tests should be considered, depending on the antibody type. For example, NMDAR seropositivity in a female should prompt a more intensive search for ovarian teratoma that includes a pelvic MRI or ultrasound.

Treatment

Randomized controlled treatment trials of autoimmune dementia are unavailable, and data pertaining to treatment are mostly derived from expert opinion, large case series, and anecdotal reports. A recent study of 72 patients with suspected autoimmune dementia reported that immunotherapy improves the neurocognitive deficits in 64% of patients. The predictors of good immunotherapy outcome were subacute onset, fluctuating course, VGKC IgG, and early immunotherapy initiation.

Based on a combination of available literature and clinical experience, we outline a therapeutic approach (Figure 2.3, Table 2.3) used for a variety of autoimmune disorders that may be similarly applied to this category of patients. The treatment of an autoimmune cause of rapidly progressive cognitive decline comprises the search for (as discussed earlier) and removal of tumor, and immunotherapy. Ultimately, the treatment protocol must be individualized for the patient, dictated by antibody detection (where at least one is found), treatment response, and severity of illness.

Cancer treatment

Early cancer detection and treatment aim to achieve stabilization or improvement of the neurological symptoms, by removing the antigenic source driving the immune response. In some patients, tumor treatment alone is effective (e.g. teratoma removal in patients with NMDAR antibody). For other patients, cancer treatment may at best bring about stabilization (e.g. small cell carcinoma treatment in a patient with ANNA-1 antibody).

Immunotherapy

The type of antibody identified may predict the neurological response to immunotherapy. Detection of antibodies targeting intracellular antigens carries a poor prognosis because of the underlying immune process mediated by cytotoxic T cell mechanisms that lead to neuronal degeneration. Conversely, detection of antibodies targeting neural surface antigens portends a more favorable outcome, because the direct pathogenic effects of these antibodies mediating disease via antigenic modulation and/or blocking may be amenable to immunotherapy. The timing of immunotherapy is also important. Case series of patients with autoimmune disorders, including autoimmune dementia, have demonstrated that early immunotherapy confers a better treatment outcome than delayed therapy. Patients treated after 1 year of symptoms generally have a poor prognosis.

The immunotherapy protocol may be subdivided into acute therapy, the "diagnostic test," and chronic "maintenance" therapy. Before starting immunotherapy, baseline neuropsychiatric testing should

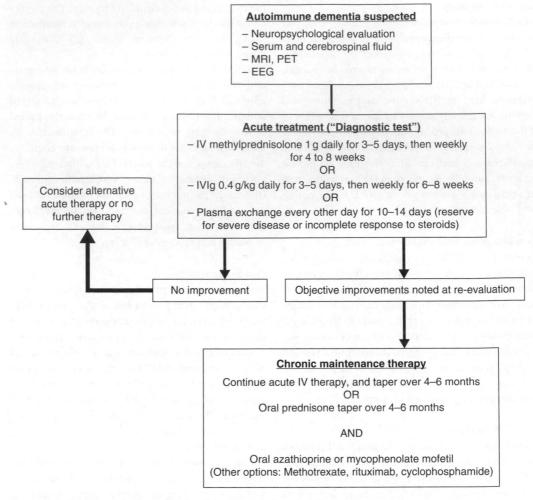

Figure 2.3 A suggested treatment algorithm for autoimmune dementias.

be performed to establish a clinical parameter for objective monitoring of immunotherapy response. Other surrogates for neurological outcome, such as antibody titers, MRI and CSF abnormalities, may be helpful as ancillary markers but should not be used as the sole parameter for measuring objective response due to unreliability.

★ **TIPS AND TRICKS**

Acute therapy – a "diagnostic test"

During the acute treatment phase, the patient's response has diagnostic implications, as a favorable response may serve as additional evidence for an autoimmune etiology. For acute

therapy, a trial of high-dose pulse intravenous corticosteroids therapy is initiated. Intravenous immunoglobulin (IVIg) is an alternative to consider in patients who cannot tolerate corticosteroids or are at risk for diabetes (including GAD65 seropositive patients). Plasma exchange may be reserved for patients who do not respond to either corticosteroids or IVIg. After the initial trial of therapy, the patient should be reevaluated for objective evidence of improvement, including a neuropsychological assessment, to demonstrate an objective response to immunotherapy. In general, patients should be reevaluated within 1 week of completing a trial of therapy.

Table 2.3 Common therapies for autoimmune neurological disorders

Treatment	Dosage	Route	Common side-effects	Therapeutic phase
Methylprednisolone	500–1000 mg daily for 3–5 days, followed by weekly for 4–8 weeks	Intravenous	Insomnia, psychiatric, hyperglycemia, electrolyte imbalances, fluid retention, hypertension, peptic ulcer, Cushing's syndrome, cataracts, infection and osteoporosis. Avascular necrosis of the hip is rare but serious side-effect. Beware Addisonian crisis on rapid withdrawal of corticosteroid	Acute and chronic taper
Intravenous immunoglobulin (IVIg)	0.4/kg daily for 3–5 days, followed by weekly or 2-weekly for 6–8 weeks	Intravenous	Headache, aseptic meningitis, thromboembolic events, acute renal failure and anaphylaxis due to IgA deficiency (rare)	Acute and chronic taper
Plasma exchange	1 exchange every other day for 10–14 days	Intravenous (usually through a central line)	Hypotension, electrolyte imbalance (hypocalcemia-related perioral paresthesia). Related to central line: infection, hemorrhage, thrombosis and pneumothorax	Acute
Azathioprine	Initially 1.5 mg/kg/day, target 2.5–3 mg/kg/day (guided by 5-point MCV increase from baseline, and TPMT value)	Oral	Gastrointestinal symptoms (nausea, vomiting, diarrhea), hypersensitivity reactions, alopecia, cytopenia and hepatotoxicity. Rare complications are lymphoma and infection	Chronic
Mycophenolate mofetil	Initially 500 mg twice daily, target 1000 mg twice daily	Oral	Gastrointestinal (diarrhea, nausea, vomiting), hypertension, peripheral edema, infections, myelosuppression, lymphoma and other malignancies	Chronic
Cyclophosphamide	IV: 500–1000 mg/m^2 monthly for 3–6 months PO: 1–2 mg/kg/day	Intravenous (IV) or oral (PO)	Gastrointestinal (nausea, vomiting), alopecia, mucositis, hemorrhagic cystitis (administer Mesna prophylaxis), infertility and myelosuppression	

PO, per os; TPMT, thiopurine methyltransferase.

The "diagnostic test" is best reserved for patients in whom the outcome is uncertain, such as those without a neural antibody detected. For patients with well-defined disorders (such as those with VGKC complex or NMDAR antibody), we favor 5 days of IV methylprednisolone (1000 mg each dose) followed by 1 mg/kg/day of oral prednisone for 3 months (while an oral steroid-sparing agent is started; see Chronic therapy below) followed by taper by 10 mg per month. Plasma exchange is reserved for patients with severe disorders or those only partially responsive to steroids. For patients with NMDAR antibody encephalitis, immunotherapy with cyclophosphamide, rituximab or both has been shown to be effective in the acute setting when first-line treatments (steroids, IVIg, and plasma exchange) have not brought about improvements. Recovery may be slow in these patients, and prolonged hospitalization and rehabilitation should be anticipated. In particular, patients who had no detectable ovarian teratoma may require more aggressive immunotherapy.

For patients with antibodies targeting intracellular antigens, such as ANNA-1, results from immunotherapy are variable but improvements are generally not dramatic. Intravenous corticosteroids and IVIg may stabilize the neurological symptoms. If neurological symptoms persist despite oncological treatment, intravenous cyclophosphamide (given as one IV pulse per month for 6 months or daily oral therapy for 6–12 months) could be considered in those with limited stage cancer, complete cancer remission, short duration of neurological symptoms, and a good oncological performance status.

Chronic therapy

If objective assessments clearly establish neurocognitive response to initial immunotherapeutic measures, chronic "maintenance" immunosuppressive therapy should be considered to maintain remission and reduce glucocorticoid or IVIg dependence. In general, azathioprine or mycophenolate mofetil are the agents of choice, having been used in a wide range of autoimmune neurological diseases. Alternatives include methotrexate, hydroxychloroquine, and oral cyclophosphamide.

The initiation of a chronic oral agent should overlap with gradual taper of corticosteroids or IVIg infusions over a period of approximately 6–8 months. This may be done by gradually extending the interval between each infusion (for example, weekly for 2 months, fortnightly for 2 months then monthly for 2 months before discontinuation). Clinical relapses can occur in up to 77% of patients during rapid immunotherapy taper or discontinuation. The tendency for relapses to occur has been reported in patients with NMDAR, AMPAR, and VGKC antibody-associated encephalitis. The patient should be closely monitored for recurrence of symptoms that occur just prior to the next infusion, which may indicate that the steroid or IVIg taper needs to be slowed down. This approach permits the oral immunosuppressants with slow onset of effect, especially azathioprine, to take effect before the infusion medications are fully discontinued. Some patients may never be able to fully wean off corticosteroid or IVIg without recrudescence of neurological symptoms. In these patients, a low dose of oral prednisolone (10–20 mg/day or every other day) may be required.

Careful monitoring for side-effects of long-term immunotherapy is crucial. This should include monitoring of blood counts, liver, and renal function. If azathioprine is the oral agent of choice, thiopurine methyltransferase (TPMT) deficiency should be excluded prior to initiation. Experience from use of azathioprine in patients with neuromyelitis optica (NMO) suggests that monitoring for a rise of mean corpuscular volume (MCV) of at least 5 points from baseline measurement is a good and reliable indicator to ensure optimum efficacy.

✋ CAUTION

Patients on glucocorticoids should also ensure a calcium intake of 1500 mg/day and vitamin D intake of 1000 IU/day, either through diet or supplements, as reduced bone mineral density may commence within the first 3 months of steroid use. Baseline and serial screening of bone density and the use of bisphosphonate treatment should be considered in patients who require longer term glucocorticoid treatment. As prophylaxis against *Pneumocystis carinii* pneumonia (PCP), trimethoprim/sulfamethoxazole is advised in patients on chronic corticosteroid or azathioprine treatment, on a regime of one double-strength table three times per week. Alternatives for sulpha-allergic patients include daily oral dapsone or monthly inhaled pentamidine.

The duration of chronic immunotherapy is not established due to lack of available data. Cases of relapses as well as spontaneous remissions have been reported. In our practice, trial of withdrawal of chronic therapy may be considered after 3–5 years of immunotherapy, depending on several factors including patient neurological improvement and lack of relapses.

Vascular causes of rapidly progressive dementia

For the most part, stroke-like deteriorations will be a feature of a vascular cause for RPD; stroke-like symptoms rarely occur in CJD and autoimmune encephalopathies. The progression may have the classical stepwise decline of vascular dementia, but often the time-course is indistinguishable from other causes of RPD. Additional helpful clinical clues include a family history of stroke and dementia, a history of recurrent stroke and migraine (cerebral autosomal dominant arteriopathy with subcortical infarcts and leukoencephalopathy [CADASIL]; Figure 2.2g,h); a history of vision loss and hearing loss (Susac syndrome); a history of malignancy (hyperviscosity syndrome).

Head MRI will likely provide more specific diagnostic clues. Basic findings include multiple strokes in the anatomical distribution of particular cerebral vessels, or multiple small vessel subcortical infarcts. Additional findings may provide clues to a specific vascular diagnosis. Hyperintensity on diffusion-weighted imaging provides insight into recent stroke events. Leptomeningeal enhancement post gadolinium contrast administration may provide additional clues for a vasculitic disorder or an autoimmune endotheliopathy (Susac disease). Similar to autoimmune dementias, early treatment of the latter two inflammatory (possibly autoimmune, but without definitive serological markers) disorders is important. A combination of corticosteroids and cyclophosphamide is the mainstay of treatment for CNS vasculitis. The approach to the treatment of Susac disease is similar to that outlined for autoimmune dementias. Distribution of abnormalities is important also. For example, diffuse areas of small vessel infarction, with involvement of white matter anterior to the temporal horns, would be suspicious for CADASIL. Small artery narrowing and beading on magnetic resonance angiography or catheter-based angiographic studies are also characteristic of vasculitis. Other unusual small vessel disorders which may present as a RPD and may be detected by MRI and basic laboratory studies include thrombotic thrombocytopenic purpura, polycythemia or other hyperviscosity syndromes.

An undetected subdural hemorrhage should always be suspected in a patient with rapid cognitive decline (usually elderly) with a history of falls leading to head injury, particularly if taking anticoagulation therapy. Elderly patients with amyloid angiopathy may present with recurrent small intracerebral hemorrhages leading to rapid cognitive decline and other neurological presentations. Again, MRI imaging is critical in these patients; characteristic findings are multiple small areas of T2 hypointensity, best observed on gradient echo (T2* or susceptibility-weighted imaging), which represent areas of hemosiderin deposition from previous hemorrhage. Anticoagulant medications should generally be avoided in these patients. At biopsy, some patients have features of both vasculitis and amyloid angiopathy. Intracranial dural arteriovenous fistula has been rarely reported as a cause of RPD.

Infectious causes of rapidly progressive dementia

Viral

Untreated HIV infection can culminate in a RPD of subcortical type. Acute onset is more often seen in the setting of seroconversion or in patients who have undergone immune reconstitution syndrome. Rarely, HIV vasculopathy can cause a RPD with strokes. A patient with progressive multifocal leukoencephalopathy can present with RPD, although progressive focal neurological signs are more common. The setting for JC virus infection is deficiency or aberrant function of T lymphocytes, the causes of which include HIV infection, immunosuppressive medication (including natalizumab in multiple sclerosis patients), and hereditary or acquired immunodeficiency states.

Viral encephalitides (including herpes – simplex, zoster, and human herpes virus 6) typically present with rapidly progressive encephalopathy leading to obtundation within days, rather than weeks to months. Subacute sclerosing panencephalitis (SSPE) is a fatal, progressive degenerative disease of the central nervous system. Affected patients are usually less than 20 years and become ill 7–10 years after initial measles infection. Conventional neuroimaging may be normal, but metabolic abnormalities may be seen on PET and SPECT imaging. Characteristic EEG findings include bursts of high-voltage complexes of 2–3 per second delta waves and sharp waves, with each complex lasting 0.5–3 sec, occurring every 3–20 sec. Each complex is followed by a relatively flat pattern. The diagnosis is made by detecting measles IgM and IgG antibodies in serum and CSF.

Bacterial

Cognitive dysfunction is a late complication of syphilis, and is sometimes rapidly progressive. Screening tests include syphilis IgG and IgM antibodies, and rapid plasma reagin (RPR) on serum, and VDRL testing on CSF. Lyme disease is a rare cause of RPD. Cognitive dysfunction is the most common manifestation of CNS Whipple's disease (caused by *T. whipplei*, a gram-positive bacillus related to Actinomycetes). Two findings are considered pathognomonic (but rare) for CNS Whipple's disease: oculomasticatory myorhythmia and oculo-facial-skeletal myorhythmia. These abnormalities are almost always accompanied by supranuclear vertical gaze palsy. A variety of other neurological findings have been described, including cerebellar ataxia, myoclonus, hemiparesis, peripheral neuropathy, seizures, and upper motor neuron disorders. Arthralgias, weight loss, diarrhea, and abdominal pain are systemic clues to the diagnosis. Isolated CNS disease in the absence of the pathognomonic findings may be difficult to recognize, since brain imaging and CSF findings are usually non-specific. Thus, one should have a low threshold for testing since this disorder is treatable with antibiotics. The diagnosis is made by identification of periodic acid-Schiff (PAS)-positive inclusions or *T. whipplei* in foamy macrophages on jejunal biopsy, or by *T. whipplei* polymerase chain reaction (PCR) of jejunal tissue or CSF.

Fungal, parasitic, and mycobacterial

Both fungal and parasitic infections may be identified as causes of RPD. Fungal agents include, in decreasing frequency, coccidioides, aspergillus, and cryptococcus. Antibody testing, fungal stains, PCR testing, and cultures of serum and CSF may

identify these patients antemortem. Severe necrotizing eosinophilic meningoencephalitis may be consistent with parasitic infection. Mycobacterial infection (*Mycobacterium neoaurum* meningoencephalitis) has rarely been reported as a cause of RPD.

Neoplastic causes of rapidly progressive dementia

Primary CNS lymphoma, intravascular lymphoma, leptomeningeal disease (lymphomatosis or carcinomatosis), and glioma may present as RPD. Often, the diagnosis should be obvious with MRI and targeted biopsy, although brain metastases, as well as the above-mentioned neoplasms, have been reportedly mistaken for CJD, with diagnosis only made at autopsy.

A major risk factor for primary CNS lymphoma (Figure 2.2b,c) is immunosuppression (HIV, medication related or congenital). Approximately 40% of patients with primary cerebral (non-Hodgkin) lymphoma present with neuropsychiatric symptoms including personality change, irritability, amnesia, confusion, language difficulty, and psychosis. MRI brain may demonstrate large solitary or multifocal T2 mildly hyperintense lesions. Periventricular lesions (including thalamic, basal ganglial, and corpus callosal lesions) are most common followed by lobar lesions. Sometimes patients may have a slowly evolving leukoencephalopathic picture (lymphomatosis cerebri) which demonstrates little or no enhancement. The CSF analysis should include cell counts, protein and glucose measurements, cytology, flow cytometry, and possibly immunoglobulin heavy-chain gene rearrangement studies by polymerase chain reaction. Imaging of spinal cord and lumbosacral nerve roots may identify a lymphomatous lesion more safely amenable to biopsy.

Intravascular lymphoma is caused by proliferation of clonal lymphocytes within blood vessels, with little or no parenchymal disease. Patients may present with a similar rapidly progressive neuropsychiatric symptom complex with or without stroke-like symptoms. Constitutional ("B") symptoms occur in the majority. MRI may demonstrate multiple areas of T2-weighted hyperintensity with patchy enhancement on T1 imaging. CSF findings may be non-specific, and biopsy of a brain lesion demonstrating T2 signal abnormality on MRI is almost always needed; the diagnosis is frequently only made at autopsy.

Gliomatosis cerebri is a rare brain neoplasm whose characteristic feature is diffuse infiltration of malignant glial cells throughout multiple central nervous system regions. Symptoms vary considerably, but a RPD phenotype is possible. Rapidly growing benign CNS tumors (such as meningiomas; Figure 2.2d) may rarely present as RPD.

Toxic causes of rapidly progressive dementia

Exposure to neurotoxins such as carbon monoxide, heavy metals (arsenic, mercury, aluminum, lithium, lead), drugs of abuse (toluene, alcohol, heroin), and therapeutic drugs (tacrolimus, cyclosporin A and some chemotherapeutic agents, such as methotrexate) can cause a rapid loss of cognitive function, but generally these patients present with an encephalopathy (over hours to days) rather than as a RPD (over weeks to months). Bismuth intoxication, typically caused by overdosing on bismuth-containing products for gastrointestinal disorders, can cause a disorder mimicking CJD. Patients initially manifest with apathy, ataxia, headaches, myoclonus, dysarthria, altered sensorium, hallucinations, and seizures. The disorder is reversible with identification and discontinuation of toxin ingestion. Extremely prolonged use can result in permanent tremors. Cranial irradiation can produce a rapidly progressive leukoencephalopathic dementia either at the time of treatment or later on (Figure 2.2e,f). Patients with multiple sclerosis are particularly prone to a rapidly progressive leukoencephalopathic course after brain irradiation.

Psychiatric causes of rapidly progressive dementia

Psychiatric disorders can sometimes mimic RPD. Pseudodementia, due to depression, may occur in a patient with a history of major depression. There are usually signs that the patient is severely depressed and decreased effort is a characteristic finding on bedside cognitive or neuropsychiatric evaluations. Many of the features of patients with true dementia may be seen in personality disorders, conversion disorders, and malingerers. The opposite is also true; psychiatric features may be an early symptom of many neurodegenerative conditions, including

CJD. Thus, a careful multidisciplinary evaluation by neurology, psychiatry, and neuropsychology specialists may be required.

Metabolic causes of rapidly progressive dementia

Comprehensive basic laboratory testing should be undertaken in any patient presenting with a RPD to exclude thyroid disease (thyroid-stimulating hormone – TSH), vitamin B12 deficiency (vitamin B12, methylmalonic acid, and homocysteine), folate deficiency, major organ failure (renal and liver function tests), and hyperparathyroidism (ionized calcium and phosphate followed by parathyroid hormone if necessary). In patients presenting with a rapidly progressive amnestic disorder in the setting of alcohol abuse (sometimes accompanied by ataxia and ophthalmoparesis, a triad known as Wernicke's encephalopathy), gastrointestinal disease (such as intractable vomiting), or suspected anorexia nervosa, thiamine deficiency needs to be strongly considered. Pellagra, a triad of dementia, dermatitis and diarrhea (due to niacin deficiency), can also arise in nutritionally deficient patients. Striatopallidonigral hypointensity on head CT is a clue to extensive cerebral calcification as a cause of neurological dysfunction, including familial disorders (Fahr's disease) and metabolic disturbances, in particular hypoparathyroidism (Fahr's syndrome).

Rarer metabolic disorders that may present as a RPD include the adult form of neuronal ceroid lipofuscinosis (Kuf's disease), Niemann Pick type C, and porphyria. Kuf's disease is an autosomal recessive lysosomal storage disease in which acid phosphatase-staining ceroid and lipofuscins accumulate in neurons, causing a progressive encephalopathy. Kuf's disease typically presents in early adulthood. Phenotypes include progressive myoclonic epilepsy, and RPD often preceded by catatonia and psychosis. Diagnosis can be established by acid phosphatase staining of ceroid and lipofuscins. The adult form of Niemann Pick type C can present acutely, and may even have a relapsing course. The most common features in addition to cognitive disorders are cerebellar ataxia, vertical supranuclear ophthalmoplegia, dysarthria, movement disorders, splenomegaly, psychiatric disorders, and dysphagia.

Table 2.4 Details regarding leukodystrophies and their evaluation

Disease	Inheritance	Clinical features	Distinct imaging features	Diagnostic tests
Adrenoleukodystrophy	X-linked recessive	Behavioral change, progressive spastic paraparesis	Posterior predominant, contrast enhancement, corticospinal tract involvement	Plasma very long chain fatty acids; ABCD1 mutation
Metachromatic leukodystrophy	Autosomal recessive	Behavioral changes, pyramidal signs, ataxia	Diffuse white matter abnormalities, with sparing of U-fibers	Arylsulfatase A in leukocytes; high urinary excretion of sulfatides
Alexander disease	Autosomal dominant in some; *de novo* mutations in others	Dementia, seizures, ataxia, bulbar symptoms	Diffuse white matter abnormalities, often anterior predominant	GFAP mutation
Leukodystrophy with neuroaxonal spheroids	Usually sporadic	Progressive dementia	Symmetrical confluent or multifocal white matter signal abnormalities	Neuroaxonal spheroids on brain biopsy
Orthochromatic leukodystrophies (heterogeneous unknown etiologies)	Sporadic or autosomal dominant	Rapidly progressive dementia	Various	Heterogeneous, unknown

Movement disorders (dystonia, parkinsonism, chorea) are more frequent than in the juvenile form. Diagnostic testing requires living cells and thus a skin fibroblast culture. Testing should be conducted in specialized centers. The "filipin test" is the most sensitive and specific diagnostic test. Fibroblasts are cultured in a low-density lipoprotein (LDL)-enriched medium, then fixed and stained with filipin (a compound forming specific complexes with unesterified cholesterol); fluorescence microscopy reveals numerous strongly fluorescent (cholesterol-filled) perinuclear vesicles. The usual acute relapsing course of acute intermittent porphyria should stand out from a RPD.

Neuropsychiatric manifestations of acute intermittent porphyria include apathy, anxiety, agitation, depression, and hallucinations. Measurement of urinary porphobilinogen is an adequate screening test in a symptomatic patient. If a screening test for increased urinary porphobilinogen is negative on spot urine testing but the index of suspicion is high, a 24-h urine collection should be obtained for quantitative assessment of delta-aminolevulinic acid, porphobilinogen, and total porphyrins.

Mitochondrial disorders

Although CNS manifestations of mitochondrial disorders are classically described as encephalopathy, often fluctuating, this disorder may be mistaken for a RPD. Additional disorders that may provide clues to a mitochondrial diagnosis include a seizure disorder, ataxia, migrainous symptoms, and psychiatric symptoms as well as one or more of deafness, retinitis pigmentosa, cardiomyopathy, diabetes mellitus, renal disorders, myopathies, and neuropathies. Measurements in CSF or muscle of lactate and pyruvate (including calculating the lactate:pyruvate ratio) and exercise testing (demonstrating a reduction in whole-body oxygen consumption and a deficit in peripheral oxygen extraction) are helpful screening tests. Further helpful diagnostic tests include identification of characteristic histochemical abnormalities (of respiratory chain function) in skin fibroblasts or muscle, and muscle histological features (subsarcolemmal and intermyofibrillar accumulation of mitochondria visualized on Gomori trichrome stain, aka "ragged red fibers"). Genetic analysis of blood, urine or muscle specimens should be performed to identify the precise genetic diagnosis.

Leukodystrophies

Many of the inherited leukodystrophies can arise acutely in adulthood, precipitated by trauma, toxins or infection (Table 2.4). Rate of progression is variable, and thus a hereditary disorder should be considered in the differential diagnosis when leukodystrophic radiological findings are observed in an adult patient with RPD. Some of the more common diagnostic considerations are listed in Table 2.4. Clinical features are usually those of a subcortical dementia (impaired attention and forgetfulness, psychomotor slowing, impaired executive and visuospatial skills, changes in personality, and emotional disturbances). A variety of clinical clues and MRI patterns of involvement may assist diagnosis or direct a more refined evaluation. For a more comprehensive review of this topic the reader is encouraged to read Costelloe et al. (2009) (see Further reading).

When to consider brain biopsy

The need to perform biopsy to secure a diagnosis has reduced over time largely due to the availability of serological/CSF markers specific for autoimmune disorders, and also neurodegenerative disorders (for example, a low CSF Abeta 42 and MRI imaging demonstrating atrophy and no signal change might indicate an atypical AD presentation). Recent experience with diffusion-weighted MRI imaging has also improved detection of CJD in atypical cases without the need for biopsy. In many cases, such as suspected neoplasm, infection or inflammatory disease, where the affected area can be visualized on MRI, a targeted biopsy can be performed if other tests have not clearly established a diagnosis. The use of blind biopsy for evaluation of dementia is controversial, as there are attendant risks for CJD transmission from infected instruments and image guidance systems.

Conclusion

Rapidly progressive dementia should be evaluated in an expedited and comprehensive manner since many disorders, previously assumed to be degenerative, have an autoimmune, inflammatory or infectious cause, and thus are potentially treatable, particularly if a diagnosis is made at an early stage.

Further reading

Castillo P, Woodruff B, Caselli R, et al. Steroid-responsive encephalopathy associated with auto-immune thyroiditis. *Arch Neurol* 2006; **63**: 197–202.

Chitravas N, Jung RS, Kofskey DM, et al. Treatable neurological disorders misdiagnosed as Creutzfeldt–Jakob disease. *Ann Neurol* 2011; **70**: 437–44.

Costello DJ, Eichler AF, Eichler FS. Leukodystrophies: classification, diagnosis, and treatment. *Neurologist* 2009; **15**: 319–28.

Dalmau J, Gleichman AJ, Hughes EG, et al. Anti-NMDA-receptor encephalitis: case series and analysis of the effects of antibodies. *Lancet Neurol* 2008; **7**: 1091–8.

Flanagan EP, McKeon A, Lennon VA, et al. Autoimmune dementia: clinical course and predictors of immunotherapy response. *Mayo Clinic Proc* 2010; **85**: 881–97.

Gaig C, Valldeoriola F, Gelpi E, et al. Rapidly progressive DLBD. *Mov Disord* 2011; **26**: 1316–23.

Geschwind MD, Shu H, Haman A, Sejvar JJ, Miller BL. RPD. *Ann Neurol* 2008; **64**: 97–108.

Josephs KA, Ahlskog JE, Parisi JE, et al. Rapidly progressive neurodegenerative dementias. *Arch Neurol* 2009; **66**: 201–7.

Kelley BJ, Boeve BF, Josephs KA. Rapidly progressive young-onset dementia. *Cogn Behav Neurol* 2009; **22**: 22–7.

Lancaster E, Martinez-Hernandez E, Dalmau J. Encephalitis and antibodies to synaptic and neuronal cell surface proteins. *Neurology* 2011; **77**: 179–89.

McKeon A, Pittock SJ. Paraneoplastic encephalomyelopathies: pathology and mechanisms. *Acta Neuropathol* 2011; **122**: 381–400.

McKeon A, Lennon VA, Pittock SJ. Immunotherapy-responsive dementias and encephalopathies. Continuum Lifelong Learning Neurol 2010; **16**: 80–101.

Schmidt C, Wolff M, Weitz M, Bartlau T, Korth C, Zerr I. Rapidly progressive AD. *Arch Neurol* 2011; **68**: 1124–30.

Vitali P, Maccagnano E, Caverzasi E, et al. Diffusion-weighted MRI hyperintensity patterns differentiate CJD from other rapid dementias. *Neurology* 2011; **76**: 1711–19.

3

Young Onset Dementia: How Much Diagnostic Testing is Enough?

Anahita Adeli and Keith A. Josephs

Divisions of Behavioral Neurology and Movement Disorders, Department of Neurology, Mayo Clinic, USA

Introduction

Dementing illnesses have a tremendous economic impact on society and healthcare in addition to considerable financial costs to families. When a young individual is afflicted with dementia there is also a substantial lost opportunity to earn income as well as decrease in workforce participation by caregivers. Family discord and negative psychological effects on the caregiver are additional difficulties. An aggressive pursuit of the underlying etiology should be initiated. That endeavor can come at a high price and therefore, a systematic and cost-efficient method must be applied.

Epidemiology

The term young onset dementia (YOD) has traditionally been used to describe a heterogeneous group of dementing disorders that affect individuals younger than 65 years of age. Few data exist on the true incidence and prevalence of all-cause dementia among persons in this age group in the United States. In a population-based study conducted in the US, the incidence rate of dementia was 8.8, 22.9, and 125.9 cases per 100,000 person-years in age groups 40–69 years, 50–59 years, and 60–64 years, respectively. Epidemiological studies of various international populations have estimated prevalence rates of 54–81 cases per 100,000 person-years. Overall, there seems to be a trend for men to be overrepresented among this population of patients. The relative frequency of YOD among all dementia patients evaluated in memory disorder clinics or tertiary referral centers varies between 6.9% and 44% depending on the city and catchment area.

> ⭑ **TIPS AND TRICKS**
>
> A number of factors can complicate and delay the diagnosis of the patient with YOD, including atypical presentations of common diseases, overlapping phenotypes of multiple different pathologies, and intrafamilial variable phenotypic expression of hereditary disorders.

Atypical presentations of common diseases can complicate and delay the diagnosis of the patient with YOD. At the same time, multiple pathologies share overlapping phenotypes. Individuals with YOD are also more likely to be misdiagnosed as having a primary psychiatric disease. Due to a combination of factors, the duration from onset of symptoms to referral is significantly longer than that for persons with late onset dementia (LOD). A wide range of pathologies exist for the underlying cause of YOD, including neurodegenerative disorders, vascular diseases, autoimmune and inflammatory diseases, infections, toxin exposure, and adult onset mitochondrial, storage, and metabolic disorders. As in LOD, neurodegenerative disorders account for the etiology in the majority of patients with EOD; however, young individuals with dementia are also more likely than elderly individuals to have a familial or non-degenerative cause.

Approach to diagnosis

The etiology of dementia in a young individual should be pursued using a standardized clinical approach (Figure 3.1). The clinical evaluation begins with obtaining a detailed history from the patient and a reliable informant regarding the nature of cognitive and behavioral symptoms, rate of decline, and evolution of symptoms over time. A thorough inquiry of any accompanying medical or neurological symptoms should be included. A review of the patient's medical history should include any history of malignancy, autoimmune disease, diabetes mellitus, cardiomyopathy, or conduction defect. The patient should be questioned about history of head injury, seizures, hearing loss, visual impairment including cataracts, weight loss, or change in bowel habits. History of tobacco use, illicit drug or alcohol use, travel, and

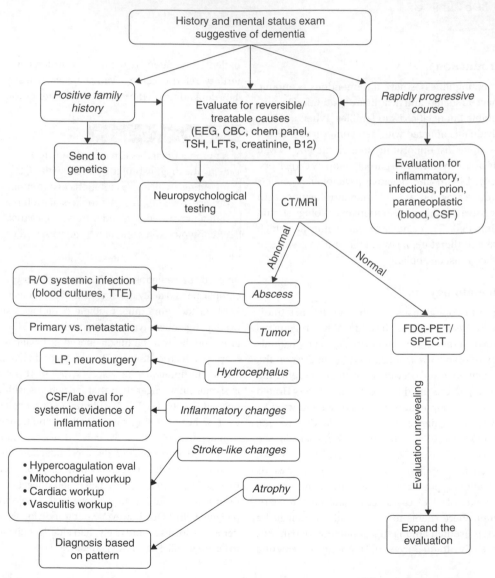

Figure 3.1 Recommendations for a staged approach to the evaluation of a patient with young onset dementia.

exposure to heavy metals, solvents or inhalants should be addressed. It is important to review performance in school, history of a learning disability, educational attainment, and occupation.

> ⚠ **CAUTION**
>
> At times a negative family history can be misleading if a family member with the mutation in question has died before the onset of neurological symptoms, the family history is being disguised for personal reasons, in adoptions or in the case of a sporadic mutation.

A family history of a dementia syndrome and/or other neurological symptoms should be aggressively explored in all patients with YOD, keeping in mind that phenotypes of a disorder may be variable within a family. A complete family history should be collected, paying attention to members with cognitive impairment or dementia, parkinsonism, motor neuron disease, mental retardation or developmental delay, stroke, death at young age, seizure disorder, psychiatric disease, autoimmune disease, or malignancy. At times a negative family history can be misleading if a family member with the mutation in question has died before the onset of neurological symptoms or in the case of a sporadic mutation. Table 3.1 provides a summary of some familial disorders that can present with YOD as well as possible co-existing neurological and medical symptoms and signs.

During the diagnostic evaluation, the physician should meet with the patient and family regularly to readdress their goals and reassess how extensive an evaluation they would like to pursue. Families should be aware that arriving at a diagnosis may provide information for the offspring of a patient with YOD in whom a genetic disorder is highly suspected and could, therefore, influence their decision about future children.

Diagnostic testing

Round 1

The rapidity of symptom onset can help to narrow the differential diagnosis. Precipitous decline in cognition often indicates an underlying vascular or infectious process affecting the central nervous system, or an acute toxic or metabolic insult. Initial laboratory studies must include a complete blood count, electrolytes, blood urea nitrogen, creatinine, liver function tests, ammonia, thyroid function tests, and toxicology screen. Emergency evaluation with neuroimaging to exclude an ischemic infarct, intracranial hemorrhage, meningitis, encephalitis, or vasculitis is mandatory. If neuroimaging and laboratory studies do not identify a cause for the acute change, a lumbar puncture to evaluate for evidence of infection or inflammation is necessary and empiric treatment with antimicrobials must be seriously considered based on the clinical circumstance. If initial lumbar puncture results (i.e. cell count, protein, and glucose) do not suggest the presence of a central nervous system (CNS) infection, an electroencephalogram (EEG) ought to be performed to rule out non-convulsive status epilepticus. If this work-up is unrevealing, then frequently neuroimaging, cerebrospinal (CSF) exam, and/or EEG may need to be repeated. Prolonged EEG monitoring may also be considered.

An insidious rate of cognitive and functional decline has a much broader differential. Epidemiological studies on cohorts of patients with YOD have identified a variety of pathological substrates (Table 3.2). A comprehensive and meticulous general and neurological examination can guide the physician in the proper direction. Special attention should be given to the presence or absence of oculomotor abnormalities, pyramidal signs, parkinsonism, dystonia, chorea, myoclonus, cerebellar signs, peripheral neuropathy, or fasciculations.

Diagnostic studies are performed to identify neurodegenerative and non-neurodegenerative causes of cognitive decline, often with the hope that a treatable etiology will be identified. The evaluation of the patient with a dementia syndrome should proceed in a thoughtful, stepwise manner in order to be efficient, conscientious of costs, and thorough while keeping in mind the wishes of the patient. The initial investigations should evaluate for treatable etiologies followed by a focused approach based on the differential generated after clinical history and examination. There are times when the initial studies do not identify the underlying etiology but the abnormalities serve to narrow the differential. If these attempts are fruitless then the differential must expand and the diagnostic evaluation should become more comprehensive.

Table 3.1 Familial disorders that can present with young onset dementia

Disorder	Most common mode of inheritance	Possible additional neurological symptoms and signs	Associated medical features	Genes most commonly identified	Comments
Alzheimer's disease	Autosomal dominant	Psychiatric disturbances, spastic paraparesis, seizures, myoclonus, ataxia, parkinsonism, dystonia, aphasia	None	*APP, PSEN1, PSEN2*	Mutations in *PSEN1* and *APP* are associated with a younger age of onset than mutations in *PSEN2*. There can be significant phenotypic heterogeneity between and within kindreds
Frontotemporal lobar degeneration	Autosomal dominant	Parkinsonism, motor neuron disease, aphasia, psychiatric disease	None	*MAPT, GRN, C9ORF72*	Clinical phenotype associated with *GRN* mutations is highly heterogeneous. Imaging often reveals focal, asymmetrical atrophy involving the frontal and/or temporal regions in symptomatic *GRN* mutation carriers whereas *MAPT* mutation carriers have a more symmetrical pattern of atrophy
Inclusion body myopathy associated with Paget disease and frontotemporal dementia	Autosomal dominant	Proximal and distal muscle weakness, psychiatric symptoms, motor neuron disease	Paget's disease of bone involving the skull, spine, and pelvis; elevated alkaline phosphatase	*VCP*	Patients are more likely to present with myopathy than cognitive impairment or Paget's disease
Parkinson's disease/Lewy body disease	Autosomal dominant/ autosomal recessive	Parkinsonism, foot dystonia, reduction of NREM or REM sleep, REM sleep behavior disorder, visual hallucinations, delusions	Dysautonomia, constipation	*SNCA, LRRK2, PRKN*	Response to levodopa is variable

Disorder	Inheritance	Clinical features	Gene	Laboratory and imaging findings
Aceruloplasminemia	Autosomal recessive	Parkinsonism, dyskinesia, dysarthria, chorea, ataxia, gait disturbance, psychiatric disease	Diabetes mellitus, hypochromic microcytic anemia, retinal degeneration	CP	Serum studies demonstrate undetectable ceruloplasmin, low copper and iron concentrations, and high serum ferritin concentration. MRI shows pattern of iron accumulation best seen on gradient echo sequences involving the striatum, thalamus, dentate nucleus and to a lesser extent, the cerebral and cerebellar cortices. Iron accumulates in the liver, but cirrhosis is not seen
Neuroferritinopathy	Autosomal dominant	Asymmetrical movement disorder, chorea, parkinsonism, focal onset dystonia	None	FTL1	Serum ferritin level is usually low, but may be normal, especially in premenopausal women. MRI shows a pattern of iron deposition best visualized on gradient echo sequences involving the red nuclei, substantia nigra and globus pallidi and to a lesser degree the dentate nuclei, thalami, basal ganglia, and precentral gyrus
Pantothenate kinase-associated neurodegeneration	Autosomal recessive	Dystonia, dysarthria and other speech disturbances, psychiatric disturbances, choreoathetosis, parkinsonism, spasticity	Pigmentary retinal degeneration	PANK2	MRI typically shows "eye of the tiger" appearance due to T2 hyperintensities in the central portion of bilateral globus pallidi surrounded by T2 hypointensity
Chorea-acanthocytosis	Autosomal recessive	Chorea, dystonia, dysphagia, dysarthria, seizures, myopathy, mild oculomotor abnormalities, psychiatric symptoms	None	VPS13A	Acanthocytes may be seen on peripheral blood smear. Elevated CK is common. MRI may show T2 hyperintensities involving the caudate and putamen, and caudate atrophy

(Continued)

Table 3.1 (*Cont'd*)

Disorder	Most common mode of inheritance	Possible additional neurological symptoms and signs	Associated medical features	Genes most commonly identified	Comments
Wilson's disease	Autosomal recessive	Parkinsonism, dystonia, chorea, dysarthria, ataxia, abnormal gait, seizures, psychiatric symptoms	Liver disease, corneal deposits (Kayser–Fleischer rings), Fanconi's syndrome, gallstones, nephrolithiasis, pancreatic disease	*ATP7B*	Normal serum ceruloplasmin is found in at least 5% of individuals with neurological symptoms. Phenotypic expression can be variable within families
Huntington's disease	Autosomal dominant	Chorea, falls, dystonia, seizures, myoclonus, parkinsonism, slowing of saccades	None	*HD*	Genetic anticipation has been demonstrated. MRI may show prominent caudate atrophy
Huntington's disease-like 2	Autosomal dominant	Parkinsonism, dysarthria, rigidity, chorea, psychiatric disturbances	None	*JPH3*	Genetic anticipation has been demonstrated. Some may have acanthocytes on peripheral smear. More common in individuals of African ancestry
Familial prion disease	Autosomal dominant	Ataxia, gait disturbance, myoclonus, chorea, psychiatric disturbances, seizures	None	*PRNP*	Abnormal MRI findings and EEG findings of periodic wave complexes are more likely to be seen in familial CJD than the other forms of familial prion disease. In familial CJD, MRI may show restricted diffusion of the caudate nucleus, putamen, thalamus, and cerebral cortex
Cerebral autosomal dominant arteriopathy with subcortical infarcts and leukoencephalopathy	Autosomal dominant	Recurrent strokes or transient ischemic attacks, seizures, migraine with aura, pseudobulbar palsy, gait disturbance	None	*NOTCH3*	MRI typically shows symmetrical T2 hyperintensities involving the periventricular and deep white matter, often initially involving the anterior temporal lobes. Multiple subcortical infarcts and deep microhemorrhages may also be present

Disease	Inheritance	Clinical features	Systemic features	Gene	Notes
Familial British dementia	Autosomal dominant	Spastic tetraparesis, ataxia, seizures, headache, stroke-like episodes, brainstem symptoms, psychiatric disturbances	None	*BRI2*	MRI shows extensive T2 hyperintensities involving the white matter, typically around the occipital and frontal horns. Cerebral hemorrhage is rare
Familial Danish dementia	Autosomal dominant	Ataxia, perceptive deafness, psychiatric disturbances	Cataracts, vitreous hemorrhages, neovascular glaucoma	*BRI2*	MRI shows extensive T2 hyperintensities involving the white matter
Familial Icelandic dementia	Autosomal dominant	Seizures, headache, strokes	None	*Cystatin C*	Intraparenchymal hemorrhages may be lobar or occur in the basal ganglia
Neuronal ceroid lipofuscinoses	Autosomal recessive	Seizures, ataxia, tremor, tic, dysarthria, facial dyskinesias, psychiatric disturbances	None	*PPT1*	Consider this diagnosis in the patient with adult onset intractable generalized epilepsy
Hereditary dentatorubral-pallidoluysian atrophy	Autosomal dominant	Choreoathetosis, ataxia	None	*DRPLA*	Genetic anticipation has been demonstrated
Fragile X-associated tremor/ataxia syndrome	X-linked dominant	Gait disturbance, ataxia, kinetic tremor, parkinsonism, impaired fine motor skills, distal lower limb peripheral neuropathy, proximal lower limb weakness, dysautonomia, psychiatric disturbances	Primary ovarian insufficiency and early infertility in females	*FMR1*	Consider in grandfathers of children with fragile X syndrome. Females are less frequently affected with a much milder phenotype and without dementia. Brain MRI typically shows global atrophy and T2 hyperintensities involving the middle cerebellar peduncles
Spinocerebellar ataxia type 17	Autosomal dominant	Ataxia, dementia, chorea, dystonia, pyramidal signs, rigidity, parkinsonism, dysphagia, dysarthria, psychiatric disturbances	None	*TBP*	Genetic anticipation has been demonstrated. MRI may show atrophy involving the cerebellum, brainstem, or cerebral hemispheres

(Continued)

Table 3.1 (*Cont'd*)

Disorder	Most common mode of inheritance	Possible additional neurological symptoms and signs	Associated medical features	Genes most commonly identified	Comments
Spinocerebellar ataxia type 2	Autosomal dominant	Ataxia, dysarthria, slowed saccadic eye movements, ophthalmoparesis, chorea, pyramidal signs, neuropathy, parkinsonism, dystoni	None	*SCA2*	Genetic anticipation has been demonstrated. MRI typically shows brainstem and cerebellar atrophy
Familial encephalopathy with neuroserpin inclusion bodies	Autosomal dominant	Seizures, myoclonus, neuropsychiatric disturbances	None	*SERPINI1*	Cognitive symptoms are typical of a frontal dysexecutive syndrome
Niemann–Pick disease type C	Autosomal recessive	Ataxia, vertical supranuclear ophthalmoplegia, dysarthria, psychiatric disturbances, dysphagia, seizures, cataplexy, perceptive deafness	Splenomegaly, hepatomegaly	*NPC1, NPC2*	MRI typically shows atrophy late in the course typically in regions corresponding to symptoms
Mitochondrial encephalomyopathy, lactic acidosis, and stroke-like episodes	Maternally inherited	Sensorineural hearing impairment, ataxia, ophthalmoplegia, seizures, recurrent stroke-like episodes, weakness, migraine, psychiatric disturbances	Diabetes mellitus, hypertrophic cardiomyopathy, short stature, dysmotility, weight loss	mtDNA (*A3243G*)	Neuroimaging may reveal basal ganglia calcifications, T2 hyperintensities in the gray and subcortical white matter especially involving the occipitoparietal lobes and crossing multiple vascular territories. MR spectroscopy of the stroke-like lesions may show elevated lactic acid levels and decreased N-acetylaspartate levels
Myoclonic epilepsy with ragged red fibers	Maternally inherited	Myoclonus, seizures, ataxia, myopathy, peripheral neuropathy, sensorineural hearing loss, optic atrophy	Short stature, cardiomyopathy, Wolff-Parkinson–White syndrome, lipomas, pigmentary retinopathy	*MT-TK, MT-TL1, MT-TH, MT-TS1*	Neuroimaging may show atrophy of the globus pallidi, cerebellum, and brainstem with calcification of the basal ganglia. EEG may show generalized spike and wave discharges

Disease	Inheritance	Clinical features		Gene	Imaging/Additional findings
Pelizaeus–Merzbacher disease	X-linked recessive	Ataxia, psychiatric disturbances, autonomic dysfunction	None	PLP1	MRI typically shows symmetrical T2 hyperintense, confluent lesions involving the periventricular white matter
Vanishing white matter syndrome	Autosomal recessive	Spasticity, seizures, ataxia, psychiatric disturbances	Ovarian failure	EIF2B	Stress, infection, or minor head injury may precede the onset of symptoms or may be associated with worsening symptoms. Females are more likely to be affected. MRI typically shows diffuse T1 hypointense and T2 hyperintense confluent lesions affected the white matter with cystic changes and cerebral atrophy
Krabbe's disease	Autosomal recessive	Paraplegia, hemiplegia, ataxia, dystonia, peripheral neuropathy	None	GALC	Symptomatic carriers will have significantly reduced galactocerebrosidase enzyme activity in leukocytes or cultured skin fibroblasts. MRI shows T2 hyperintensities involving the periventricular white matter with posterior predominance
Metachromatic leukodystrophy	Autosomal recessive	Seizures, psychiatric disturbances, peripheral neuropathy, spasticity, weakness, ataxia	None	ARSA, PSAP	Urinary sulfatides are elevated. MRI shows diffuse, symmetrical T2 hyperintensities involving the periventricular white matter with anterior predominance initially
Canavan's disease	Autosomal recessive	Spasticity, dystonia, seizures	None	ASPA	Individuals of Ashkenazi Jewish heritage are most affected. Urinary NAA is elevated. MRI may show diffuse subcortical T2 hyperintensities typically involving the arcuate fibers

(Continued)

Table 3.1 (*Cont'd*)

Disorder	Most common mode of inheritance	Possible additional neurological symptoms and signs	Associated medical features	Genes most commonly identified	Comments
Adrenomyeloneuropathy ± leukodystrophy	X-linked recessive	Ataxia, psychiatric disturbances, spastic paraparesis, peripheral neuropathy, sexual and sphincter dysfunction	Adrenal insufficiency, primary testicular failure, red-green color blindness	*ABCD1*	Heterozygote females have a more heterogeneous presentation, but do not develop cerebral demyelination. Elevated plasma or serum very long chain fatty acids may be present and are diagnostic. MRI shows spinal cord atrophy and symmetrical T2 hyperintensities in the periventricular region with a posterior predominance and contrast enhancement along the margin of active demyelination
Cerebrotendinous xanthomatosis	Autosomal recessive	Spasticity, cerebellar signs, dystonia, parkinsonism, peripheral neuropathy, seizures, psychiatric disturbances	Cataracts, tendon xanthomas	*CYP27A1*	MRI typically shows cerebral and cerebellar atrophy, symmetrical T2 hyperintensities involving the periventricular white matter, dentate nucleus, medial globus pallidus, substantia nigra, and inferior olive. Spinal cord MRI may show T2 hyperintensities involving the dorsolateral columns of the spinal cord. Therapy with chenodeoxycholic acid is effective
Hereditary diffuse leukodystrophy with spheroids	Autosomal dominant	Psychiatric disturbances, pyramidal signs	None	unknown	MRI typically shows T2 hyperintense and T1 hypointense symmetrical and confluent signal change involving the subcortical, deep and periventricular white matter with a frontal predominance. Sporadic forms also exist

Familial idiopathic basal ganglia calcification	Autosomal dominant (majority)	Neuropsychiatric disturbance, gait impairment, dysarthria, dysphagia, clumsiness, involuntary movements, seizures	None	unknown	Imaging shows bilateral lentiform nuclei calcification which may progress over time and also involve the caudate, thalami, and dentate nuclei, as well as cerebral white matter. Affected family members may be asymptomatic
Hereditary vitamin E deficiency	Autosomal recessive	Ataxia, loss of proprioception and vibratory sense, distal weakness, titubation, decreased visual acuity	None	*TTPA*	Plasma alpha-tocopherol is significantly reduced. MRI may show cerebellar atrophy. Treatment is with high-dose oral vitamin E supplementation
Lafora disease	Autosomal recessive	Ataxia, myoclonus, seizures	None	*EPM2A, NHLRC1*	MRI may be normal. EEG shows epileptiform discharges with occipital predominance. Skin biopsy may show periodic acid Schiff-positive intracellular inclusion bodies.

CJD, Creutzfeldt–Jakob disease; CK, creatine kinase; MRI, magnetic resonance imaging; NAA, N-acetyl aspartate; NREM, non-rapid eye movement; REM, rapid eye movement.

Table 3.2 Etiologies of dementia in cohorts of patients less than 65 years

Source	Harvey et al[1].	McMurtray et al[2].	Yokota et al[3].	Kelley et al[4].	Nandi et al[5].	Papageorgiou et al[6].	Garre-Olmo et al[7].
Location	United Kingdom	Los Angeles, California	Japan	Rochester, Minnesota	India	Greece	Spain
Setting	Community-based catchment area	Cognitive disorders clinic	Cognitive disorders clinic	Medical record linkage system	Cognitive disorders clinic	Cognitive disorders clinic	Registry of dementia cases
Number of patients	185	278	34	235	93	114	144
Males:females	107:78	270:8	NR	119:116	61:32	55:59	73:71
Mean number of years of education	NR	13.7	NR	13.9	11	9.6	7.4
Age range, years	30–64	<65	41–64	17–45	39–64	46–64	30–64
Mean age at onset, years	NR	51.5	NR	34.7	56.5	55.1	58.1
Mean age at consultation, years	58.7	56.5	NR	36.7	NR	58.7	61.3
Mean duration of symptoms prior to presentation, years	NR	NR	NR	2	3.5	3.7	3.9
Alzheimer's disease (%)	62 (33.5)	48 (17.3)	13 (38.2)	4 (1.7)	31 (33.3)	31 (27.2)	61 (42.4)
Vascular dementia (%)	34 (18.4)	80 (28.8)	8 (23.5)	7 (3.0)	19 (20.4)	7 (6.1)	20 (13.8)
Mixed Alzheimer's disease + vascular dementia	NR	NR		NR	NR	NR	9 (6.3)
Frontotemporal dementia (%)	23 (12.4)	7 (2.5)	5 (14.7)	31 (13.2)	25 (26.9)	28 (24.6)	14 (9.7)
Parkinson's disease dementia (%)	2 (1.1)	10 (3.6)*	0	1 (0.4)	4 (4.3)	2 (1.8)	3 (2.1)

Huntington disease (%)	9 (4.9)	4 (1.4)	NR	18 (7.7)	4 (4.3)	3 (2.6)	3 (2.1)
Lewy body disease (%)	12 (6.5)	NR	1 (2.9)	1 (0.4)	NR	3 (2.6)	1 (0.7)
Corticobasal degeneration (%)	2 (1.1)	1 (0.4)	0	3 (1.3)	NR	0	2 (1.4)
Progressive supranuclear palsy (%)	NR	NR	0	1 (0.4)	1 (1.1)	7 (6.1)	1 (0.7)
Multiple sclerosis (%)	8 (4.3)	8 (2.9)	NR	26 (11.1)	2 (2.2)	1 (0.9)	NR
Vasculitis (%)	NR	NR	NR	7 (3.0)	2 (2.2)	1 (0.9)	NR
Other autoimmune or inflammatory disease (%)	NR	NR	NR	24 (10.2)	NR	1 (0.9)	NR
Normal pressure hydrocephalus (%)	NR	6 (2.2)	NR	4 (1.7)	NR	1 (0.9)	NR
Infectious (including prion disease, HIV) (%)	2 (1.1)	25 (9.0)	NR	11 (4.7)	3 (3.2)	10 (8.8)	2 (1.4)
Alcohol-related dementia (%)	19 (10.3)	15 (5.4)	0	1 (0.4)	NR	NR	5 (3.5)
Metabolic disorder (%)	NR	NR	NR	25 (10.6)	NR	NR	NR
Traumatic brain injury (%)	Excluded	67 (24.1)	3 (8.8)	Excluded	NR	1 (0.9)	2 (1.4)
Other/unknown (%)	12 (6.5)/NR	7 (2.5)/NR	4 (11.8)/NR	27 (11.5)/44 (18.7)	2 (2.2)/NR	18 (15.8)/NR	21 (14.6)/NR
Positive family history (%)	NR	NR	NR	25.5	17.2	NR	34.3

*Reported as "parkinsonian disorders" including multisystem atrophy.

NR, not reported.

The initial laboratory testing should serve as a screen for infection or inflammatory conditions, metabolic abnormalities, common nutritional deficiencies, and endocrinopathies.

The complete blood count with leukocyte differential count can rapidly screen for the presence of an inflammatory state, infection, anemia, or malignancy. The presence of normocytic anemia may suggest the existence of gastrointestinal blood loss, poor nutrition, hemolysis, renal insufficiency, primary bone marrow disorder, or anemia of chronic disease, the latter including autoimmune disease, acute or chronic infection, and malignancy. Macrocytic anemia is often associated with alcohol abuse, vitamin B12 deficiency or folate deficiency, if not due to a medication effect. Marked macrocytic anemia (i.e. mean corpuscular volume >110 fL) is due to primary bone marrow disease until proven otherwise. Microcytic anemia can be evidence of iron deficiency, thalassemia, or anemia of chronic disease. Acquired neutropenia may be due to underlying infection or sepsis, drug effect, hematological malignancy, or autoimmune disease (e.g. systemic lupus erythematosus). Acquired lymphopenia can be seen with infection including that from human immunodeficiency virus (HIV), autoimmune disease, connective tissue disease, renal insufficiency, and alcohol abuse. Thrombocytosis may be due to non-myeloid or myeloid malignancy, hemolysis, infection, or chronic inflammatory state. Thrombocytopenia can be seen with thrombotic thrombocytopenic purpura, drug effect, hypersplenism, connective tissue disease, lymphoproliferative disorders, HIV infection, or idiopathic thrombocytopenic purpura.

Sedimentation rate and C-reactive protein are inflammatory markers which can be used as a nonspecific screen for malignancy, infection, autoimmune disease, or kidney disease.

Basic metabolic profile which includes electrolytes, creatinine, and blood urea nitrogen should be performed to screen for chronic renal insufficiency and electrolyte derangements. The presence of renal disease and cognitive impairment may suggest a multisystem disorder such as mitochondrial disease, systemic vasculitis (e.g. due to Wegener's granulomatosis or systemic lupus erythematosus), or sarcoidosis. Renal dysfunction due to diabetes or hypertension can be associated with cerebrovascular disease.

Hyponatremia can be a sign of cerebral salt wasting syndrome or syndrome of inappropriate antidiuretic hormone secretion as seen in a number of neurological disorders such as meningitis or encephalitis, including autoimmune or paraneoplastic limbic encephalitis related to voltage-gated potassium antibodies. Many medical conditions can also cause hyponatremia such as congestive heart failure, hepatic failure, renal disease, hypothyroidism, adrenal insufficiency, polydipsia in patients with psychiatric disease, and medication related. Hyponatremic encephalopathy is the most serious clinical manifestation of hyponatremia. The clinical manifestations may include headache, confusion, psychosis, abnormalities of gait, depressed level of consciousness, or seizures. Rapid correction of hyponatremia can result in an osmotic demyelination syndrome in which encephalopathy, parkinsonism, mutism, pseudobulbar palsy, seizures, and locked-in syndrome have all been described.

Screening for an associated endocrinopathy with thyroid function tests, parathyroid hormone, and calcium should be performed early in the diagnostic evaluation. Chronic hypocalcemia, hypothyroidism, hyperthyroidism, hypoparathyroidism, hyperparathyroidism, and hypercortisolism have all been reported to result in psychosis or dementia.

Cognitive and behavioral symptoms can be associated with vitamin B12 deficiency, even in the absence of anemia or macrocytosis, and are often accompanied by sensory loss, paresthesias, and ataxia. A frontotemporal dementia (FTD) syndrome has been described with accompanying frontoparietal and anterior temporal hypoperfusion on brain single photon emission computed tomography (SPECT), with clinical resolution of symptoms and improvement of cerebral perfusion after cyanocobalamin supplementation. If vitamin B12 deficiency is confirmed, then screening for pernicious anemia should occur, with either intrinsic factor antibodies or the Schilling test, before determining that the cause of deficiency is due to primary intestinal malabsorption.

Elevated transaminases and hyperammonemia can be associated with a hepatic encephalopathy which is characterized by altered mentation (e.g. decreased attention, amnesia, confusion) and personality changes (e.g. apathy, depression, euphoria, paranoia) or coma if severe.

Structural neuroimaging, ideally with an magnetic resonance imaging (MRI) study if not contraindicated, should be performed early in the evaluation of YOD. In addition to providing evidence of inflammatory, ischemic, or structural pathology, this can provide information regarding whether a particular pattern of atrophy is present consistent with a specific neurodegenerative disorder. Individuals with Alzheimer's disease (AD) dementia tend to have diffuse cortical atrophy with more pronounced atrophy involving the hippocampi and posterior temporoparietal lobes, whereas patients with FTD typically have symmetrical or asymmetrical volume loss predominantly affecting the frontal and anterior temporal lobes. On the other hand, dementia with Lewy bodies (DLB) is not typically associated with cortical atrophy but rather atrophy of the dorsal midbrain, substantia innominata, and hypothalamus which may be difficult to visualize on standard MRI sequences. MRI findings in progressive supranuclear palsy are best visualized in the midsagittal plane. Atrophy of the midbrain tegmentum gives a characteristic appearance of a hummingbird in progressive supranuclear palsy. Volume loss of the middle potion of the anterior corpus callosum, anterior cingulate, and frontal cortex, to a lesser degree, may also be seen. Corticobasal syndrome, whether due to corticobasal ganglionic degeneration or another pathological substrate, is typically associated with atrophy of the middle corpus callosum, superior parietal, and posterior frontal lobes.

Coronal MR images should be included as they provide an alternative view for visual inspection of medial temporal lobe structures to assess for atrophy which can be seen in AD and FTD, and also to evaluate for hippocampal sclerosis. Coronal fluid-attenuated inversion recovery (FLAIR) images are crucial in cases of suspected limbic encephalitis as this allows for optimal visualization of hyperintensities involving the medial and basal temporal lobes.

Diffusion-weighted imaging sequences ought to be performed to evaluate for the presence of acute or subacute ischemic infarcts which may be a result of arterial or venous occlusion, primary CNS vasculitis, or secondary vasculitides from infection, collagen vascular disease, or drugs. Restricted diffusion may also be seen with pyogenic abscess, acute demyelination, tumor with a high cellularity, or osmotic demyelination syndrome. Hypoglycemia, hypoxic-ischemic insult, and carbon monoxide poisoning each result in a characteristic pattern of restricted diffusion as well. Individuals with Creutzfeldt–Jakob disease (CJD) may have restricted diffusion involving the striatum, thalamus, and/or cortical ribbon.

The presence of multiple microhemorrhages detected on gradient echo MR sequences should alert the physician to possible cerebral amyloid angiopathy, which can be associated with AD, or chronic hypertension. Cerebral autosomal dominant arteriopathy with subcortical infarcts and leukoencephalopathy (CADASIL), diffuse axonal injury associated with traumatic head injury, and CNS vasculitis are less common causes of cerebral microhemorrhages. Gradient echo sequences can more easily identify brain iron deposition as can be seen in neuroferritinopathy, pantothenate kinase-associated neurodegeneration, and aceruloplasminemia. Bilateral hypointensities of the globus pallidi on gradient echo sequences are also associated with chronic hepatic encephalopathy which is felt to most likely reflect deposition of manganese and correspond to hyperintensities on T1 sequences.

White matter disease is typically best seen on FLAIR images and can present with a variety of cognitive symptoms. The differential in the young patient with dementia and an MRI consistent with a leukoencephalopathy can be quite broad and includes dysimmune, infectious, postinfectious, vascular, metabolic, nutritional, neoplastic, toxic, demyelinating, or mitochondrial disorders. Administration of contrast may help to narrow the possibilities. The adult onset leukodystrophies have a more heterogeneous presentation than the childhood forms and can present acutely or with a slowly progressive course spanning decades. Disorders of the urea cycle, fatty acid oxidation, or amino acid catabolism may present with a progressive dementing syndrome accompanied by spastic paraparesis and psychiatric disturbances often exacerbated by stressors such as minor trauma, pregnancy, or infection. These individuals may be misdiagnosed as having multiple sclerosis or a primary psychiatric disorder.

If the imaging study reveals evidence of "brain sagging" with swelling of brainstem structures and low-lying cerebellar tonsils, then additional studies such as CT myelography or heavily T2-weighted MR myelography should be pursued to rule out a CSF leak. Brain sagging has been described to cause a behavioral variant FTD phenocopy which has been referred to as frontotemporal brain sagging syndrome. Pachymeningeal enhancement should prompt further evaluation with a lumbar puncture to measure the opening pressure as low pressure can give this picture. In addition, CSF analysis to evaluate for evidence of inflammation, infection, and malignancy may be necessary.

Round 2

If the above laboratory and imaging studies are non-diagnostic and the patient and family are interested in pursuing further testing to arrive at a diagnosis, then the next round of testing should follow.

Autoimmune and collagen vascular diseases should be considered in all patients with YOD, but especially in those with onset of dementia shortly following pregnancy, family history or personal history of preexisting autoimmune disease, signs or symptoms suggestive of underlying collagen vascular disease (e.g. uveitis, arthritis, sicca syndrome, unexplained fevers, or recurrent oral or genital ulcers). Screening labs can include serum antinuclear antibody, rheumatoid factor, anti-Ro and anti-La antibodies, antiphospholipid antibodies (i.e. lupus anticoagulant, anticardiolipin antibodies, and anti-beta2-glycoprotein-1 antibodies), angiotensin converting enzyme, and autoantibodies to thyroid peroxidase and thyroglobulin. A pathergy test should be performed if Behçet's disease is being considered.

Serological testing for *Treponema pallidum*, HIV, and *Borrelia burgdorferi* should be performed early to screen for these infectious etiologies for which there are treatments.

An elevation in serum amylase can be associated with pancreatic encephalopathy which can manifest as cognitive impairment, focal neurological signs, and psychosis.

Neuropsychological assessment is a tool that can be used to demonstrate subtle cognitive impairment that may be difficult to detect on the bedside mental status exam. In addition, it can provide valuable information on the extent and severity of cognitive dysfunction. A particular pattern of cognitive impairment may become evident and assist in making the diagnosis of a specific neurodegenerative disorder.

An EEG is a non-invasive tool that in this setting may be pursued if non-convulsive status epilepticus or subclinical seizures are suspected, or in the patient with a rapidly progressive dementia. Bilateral, generalized, or unilateral periodic bi- or triphasic sharp wave complexes is a pattern suggestive of CJD in the appropriate clinical context and is typically seen in certain subtypes. Serial EEG recordings may be required if suspicion for CJD is high. Seizures, including those refractory to anticonvulsants, have been associated with paraneoplastic and non-paraneoplastic limbic encephalitis as well as a steroid-responsive encephalopathy associated with autoimmune thyroiditis. Encephalopathy is usually accompanied by slowing of the posterior dominant rhythm to a degree correlated with the extent of cortical dysfunction, but is an otherwise non-specific finding. Subacute sclerosing panencephalitis (SSPE), which is more common in underdeveloped and developing countries due to the lower rates of measles immunization, is rarely seen in adults. However, there is growing concern that its incidence will increase in developed countries in the face of possible decline in vaccination due to unconfirmed claims regarding increased risk of autism. EEG in SSPE typically shows periodic, bisynchronous, high-amplitude slow waves occurring at long repetition intervals.

An electrocardiogram can be performed as a screen for cardiomyopathy or conduction defects seen in HIV, Lyme disease, mitochondrial, lipid, and amino acid disorders. Chest x-ray can be performed to screen for lung cancer, pulmonary tuberculosis, or sarcoidosis.

Cerebrospinal fluid examination should include cell count with differential, protein, and glucose. Measurements of IgG index and oligoclonal bands should be performed in all cases to evaluate for the presence of an immunological response. Evaluation for chronic meningoencephalitis should include polymerase chain reaction (PCR) for *Tropheryma whipplei*, Lyme serology, India ink stain, culture for *Cryptococcus neoformans*, acid-fast bacilli smear and culture for tuberculosis, and PCR for herpes simplex virus type 2. An elevated level of neuron-specific enolase, 14-3-3, and/or tau is indicative of rapid neuronal death and can be used as adjunctive tests in the diagnosis of CJD. A low CSF amyloid beta $_{1-42}$ and high total tau or phosphorylated tau is suggestive of AD pathology with good sensitivity and specificity. In the immunocompromised patient, CSF analysis should include PCRs for human herpesvirus-6, human herpesvirus-7, JC virus, and cytomegalovirus. Further microbial studies should be guided by the results of neuroimaging and initial CSF studies.

Evaluating for the presence of a paraneoplastic antibody is reasonable in all patients in whom the initial work-up is unrevealing. If serum paraneoplastic antibodies are negative and clinical suspicion is high, then the CSF should be tested as there are cases in which an autoantibody may only be detected in the CSF. Testing for an occult malignancy should parallel the search for a paraneoplastic antibody. Whole-body positron emission tomography using [^{18}F] fluorodeoxyglucose (FDG-PET) has a significantly higher sensitivity than CT alone in detecting occult malignancy. A PET scan may also identify granulomatous disease. Given the cost of a whole-body PET scan, it is reasonable to begin with CTs of the chest, abdomen, and pelvis, mammography in women, prostate-specific antigen in men, and/or testicular ultrasound in young men. A transvaginal ultrasound is the preferred imaging modality for detecting primary adnexal malignancy in females, followed by an MRI with contrast if a mass is identified. The imaging studies performed may also be guided by the specific antibody detected.

Round 2.5

Alternative diagnostic studies may be necessary based on the patient's clinical presentation, co-morbidities, exam findings, or results of testing performed early in the evaluation.

For patients in whom malnutrition is suspected (e.g. those with end-stage liver or renal disease, chronic obstructive lung disease, malabsorption syndrome, alcoholism, malignancy, cystic fibrosis, short bowel syndrome, or prior bariatric surgery), in addition to electrolyte and vitamin B12 levels, screening for other nutritional deficiencies should be considered. Niacin (vitamin B3) deficiency causes a constellation of symptoms known as pellagra in which a painful dermatitis involving skin exposed to sun or pressure, diarrhea, psychiatric disturbance, and dementia are present. Measurement of erythrocyte transketolase activity can serve as an indicator of thiamine status, deficiency of which is associated with Wernicke–Korsakoff syndrome. Serum vitamin E level should

be checked as severe deficiency, whether due to acquired or familial etiologies, can present with progressive neurological deterioration marked by peripheral neuropathy, ataxia, myopathy, and dementia. Copper, retinol (vitamin A), zinc, biotin, and vitamin B6 are each rarely associated with a potentially reversible encephalopathy and serum levels should be measured in the appropriate clinical circumstance.

If neuroimaging shows evidence of previous infarcts, the underlying etiology should be identified, beginning with evaluating for typical cerebrovascular risk factors with lipid profile, fasting glucose or glycosylated hemoglobin, hypercoagulable panel, and echocardiogram. In addition to the connective tissue screening laboratory studies mentioned above, serum antineutrophil cytoplasmic antibodies and cryoglobulins may be diagnostic. An underlying mitochondrial disorder may also need to be pursued.

In the patient with an accompanying movement disorder such as chorea, parkinsonism, or dystonia, serum ferritin, copper, ceruloplasmin, and 24-h urinary copper should be measured. The peripheral blood smear can provide additional information. Acanthocytes are associated with a number of neurodegenerative disorders including chorea-acanthocytosis, Huntington's disease-like 2, and pantothenate kinase-associated neurodegeneration. A slit-lamp examination should be performed to evaluate for the presence of Kayser–Fleischer rings. The presence of ataxia should prompt measurements of serum vitamin E, vitamin B12, copper, IgA endomysial and tissue transglutaminase antibodies, and paraneoplastic antibodies.

An overnight polysomnogram can be performed if obstructive sleep apnea or rapid eye movement (REM) sleep behavior disorder is suspected. REM sleep behavior disorder has been associated with limbic encephalitis and preceding or accompanying DLB. Insomnia and narcolepsy are each also associated with limbic encephalitis.

If clinical suspicion is present, electromyogram and nerve conduction studies should be performed to evaluate for co-existing motor neuron disease, myopathy, or peripheral neuropathy.

Round 3

Functional imaging of the brain using FDG-PET is a reliable and valid diagnostic tool that can provide additional data early in the investigation to support the diagnosis of a specific neurodegenerative disorder, but should not be interpreted in isolation of the clinical picture. A pattern of hypometabolism involving the posterior temporal and posterior parietal lobes, including the posterior cingulate and precuneal regions, with sparing of the primary visual, sensory, and motor cortices, is classic for AD dementia. In FTD, hypometabolism is more often seen in anterior temporal, anterior cingulate, and frontal regions. Patients with DLB tend to have similar patterns of metabolic reductions as those of patients with AD, with significant hypometabolism involving the posterior cingulate and parietotemporal regions, but with additional hypometabolism involving the primary visual cortex. Caudate and putamen hypometabolism are seen in Huntington's disease, even in early stages.

If a mitochondrial cytopathy is suspected, then serum and CSF lactate and pyruvate should be measured, but negative results do not rule out the diagnosis. A fasting or postexercise sample of CSF and serum lactate may increase the sensitivity. Quantification of urine and plasma amino acids should identify an amino acid disorder and an elevated alanine may be suggestive of a mitochondrial cytopathy. Measurement of urine organic acids and blood spot acyl carnitines can identify an organic acid or mitochondrial disorder. Serum ammonia level should be checked to screen for a urea cycle disorder in the encephalopathic patient. An elevated creatine kinase may be indicative of a mitochondrial disorder as well.

Enzyme assays on leukocytes or cultured skin fibroblasts can also be performed to diagnose some of the lysosomal storage disorders. Accumulation of the stored material due to the enzyme defect may be measured in the tissue or urine (e.g. N-substituted amino acid in Canavan's disease and sulfatides in metachromatic leukodystrophy).

In addition to screening for possible mitochondrial or lipid storage disease in the young patient with episodic cognitive or behavioral symptoms, screening for porphyria should be considered and includes measurements of urinary porphobilinogen, ideally when the patient is symptomatic. If the screening test is negative but there is strong suspicion, further testing should proceed with quantification of porphobilinogen, delta-aminolevulinic acid, and total porphyrins from a 24-h urinary collection.

If adrenomyeloneuropathy is suspected, serum very long chain fatty acids should be measured.

Mercury, arsenic, lead, manganese, tin, thallium, and aluminum are some of the heavy metals for which chronic exposure can result in dementia. A 24-h urinary collection can be used to confirm toxicity for arsenic, mercury, thallium, or tin. Consumption of seafood should be avoided for 3 days prior to testing as it can raise urinary arsenic levels. Lead and manganese should be measured in the blood to demonstrate toxicity. Elevation in the blood level of aluminum following deferoxamine infusion is diagnostic of aluminum toxicity. Basophilic stippling of red blood cells is seen on peripheral blood smear in cases of lead, aluminum, or arsenic toxicity.

Referral to colleagues in other medical departments may be necessary to find evidence of systemic involvement of a disorder. An ophthalmological examination may provide valuable information. Optic atrophy and/or retinitis pigmentosa are associated with mitochondrial or lysosomal storage disease. Retinal degeneration, corneal clouding, and a cherry-red spot are each associated with storage diseases. Cataracts can be associated with some leukodystrophies or cerebrotendinous xanthomatosis. Ocular and optic nerve changes are seen in paraneoplastic disorders and immune-mediated disease such as Behçet's disease, sarcoidosis, and systemic lupus erythematosus. A slit-limp examination should be included to identify Kayser–Fleischer rings associated with Wilson's disease. In patients in whom metabolic or mitochondrial disorders are being considered, colleagues in pediatric neurology can be instrumental.

Round 4

★ TIPS AND TRICKS

GeneTests (www.genetests.org) is an online source for healthcare providers for up-to-date reviews of clinical syndromes, medical genetics, and the clinical and/or research laboratories where genetic tests are available.

Genetic testing may be pursued in those with a positive family history or if the patient's symptomatology is suggestive of a genetic disorder. This may be performed earlier in the evaluation depending on the level of suspicion of a specific genetic disorder. Prior genetic counseling is mandatory and should include discussions of potential risks to children and available reproductive options. If a genetic mutation is not identified and a familial disorder is strongly suspected based on the family history, a variety of genetic techniques may be employed to identify a novel disease-causing mutation within a family.

EVIDENCE AT A GLANCE

Antemortem examination of cerebral tissue results in a pathological diagnosis in 57% of patients with a dementia syndrome not typical of a neurodegenerative disorder.

When there is uncertainty regarding the diagnosis, brain biopsy may provide the diagnosis. Given the risk associated with a neurosurgical procedure, this is often reserved for patients in whom a treatable etiology is suspected based on the neuroimaging, CSF, or laboratory studies such as underlying infection, inflammatory process, malignancy, or vasculitis, rather than for those with a typical presentation of a neurodegenerative disorder. In a retrospective series, antemortem examination of cerebral tissue resulted in a pathological diagnosis in 57% of patients with a dementia syndrome not typical of a neurodegenerative disorder. Ten percent of all patients were diagnosed with a treatable illness. Brain biopsy ideally should target a lesion identified on neuroimaging such as an area of pathological enhancement of an intraparenchymal lesion, and should include the meninges, cortex, and white matter.

Biopsy of extraneural tissues is a less invasive approach that may be diagnostic in the appropriate circumstance. Biopsy of the tonsils or other lymphoreticular tissue can be diagnostic in patients with variant-CJD. The diagnosis of celiac disease or Whipple's disease may be made on small bowel biopsy. Biopsy-proven dermatitis herpetiformis is diagnostic of celiac disease as well. Electron microscopy of skin biopsy can allow for the diagnosis of lysosomal storage disorders, Lafora body disease, Sneddon syndrome, or CADASIL. Skin biopsy for fibroblast culture may be diagnostic of a mitochondrial cytopathy or Niemann-Pick type C. Nerve biopsy can identify a number of hereditary conditions such as adult polyglucosan body disease and metachromatic leukodystrophy. Labial salivary gland biopsy may confirm the presence of Sjögren's syndrome. A conjunctival biopsy is a non-invasive procedure that can be performed early in the initial evaluation of suspected sarcoidosis or Sjögren's syndrome. A muscle biopsy may be performed to evaluate for histological evidence of vasculitis, sarcoidosis, mitochondrial disease, or CADASIL. Rectal biopsy can play a role in identifying neurolipidosis, metachromatic leukodystrophy, or neuronal intranuclear inclusion disease. Bone marrow examination can aid in the diagnosis of hematological malignancy, sarcoidosis, or lipid storage diseases. Liver biopsy may be diagnostic of Lafora body disease, Wilson's disease, or a mitochondrial cytopathy.

The order in which the above investigations are considered and the extent to which particular diagnoses are pursued should be entirely guided by the patient's symptom complex, family history, physical exam, and results of testing along the way. Many cases will require extensive evaluations in order to make accurate diagnoses, whereas others will be relatively straightforward. In each case, the constellation of neurological symptoms and signs is unique and the subsequent evaluation should reflect that.

In the event of an unsuccessful diagnosis

Patients in whom the investigations are unrevealing should be followed for evolution of symptoms and changes in examination. Certain tests may need to be repeated over the course of the illness. The quest to identify the cause of a dementing illness in a young patient may be laborious and can be exhausting for the patient and family. Some of the above studies may be especially difficult for the patient with behavioral problems and this must be carefully considered before proceeding blindly. During the evaluation, regular meetings should take place to readdress the goals of the patient and family and to discuss how extensive an evaluation they are willing to undergo. It is important to discuss with them early in the diagnostic course that despite an earnest effort, an antemortem diagnosis cannot be made in a small percentage of cases. If not otherwise contraindicated, an empirical, 3–5-day trial of an intravenous corticosteroid may be considered, especially in those with a rapidly progressive course, an inflammatory appearing CSF and/or a co-existing inflammatory disorder. If a desirable response is seen, then maintenance treatments or alternative immunosuppressant therapies can be considered.

In instances in which a confident diagnosis cannot be made or when the diagnosis is not based on a positive genetic test result, the value of autopsy should be discussed openly after a sound relationship has been established with the patient and family, as identifying the cause of the dementia may have medical relevance to offspring, siblings, and more distant relatives.

Acknowledgments

KAJ is supported by NIH grants R01 DC 010367 (PI), R01 AG 037491 (PI), a Dana Foundation grant (PI) and R21 AG 38736 (Co-I).

References

[1] Harvey RJ, Skelton-Robinson M, Rossor MN. The prevalence and causes of dementia in people under the age of 65 years. *J Neurol Neurosurg Psychiatry* 2003; **74**(9): 1206–9.

[2] McMurtray A, Clark DG, Christine D, Mendez MF. Early-onset dementia: frequency and causes compared to late-onset dementia. *Dement Geriatr Cogn Disord* 2006; **21**(2): 59–64.

[3] Yokota O, Sasaki K, Fujisawa Y, et al. Frequency of early and late-onset dementias in a Japanese memory disorders clinic. *Eur J Neurol* 2005; **12**(10): 782–90.

[4] Kelley BJ, Boeve BF, Josephs KA. Young-onset dementia: demographic and etiologic characteristics of 235 patients. *Arch Neurol* 2008; **65**(11): 1502–8.

[5] Nandi SP, Biswas A, Pal S, Basu S, Senapati AK, Das SK. Clinical profile of young-onset dementia: a study from Eastern India. *Neurol Asia* 2008; 13: 103–8.

[6] Papageorgiou SG, Kontaxis T, Bonakis A, Kalfakis N, Vassilopoulos D. Frequency and causes of early-onset dementia in a tertiary referral center in Athens. *Alzheimer Dis Assoc Disord* 2009; **23**(4): 347–51.

[7] Garre-Olmo J, Genis Batlle D, del Mar Fernandez M, et al. Incidence and subtypes of early-onset dementia in a geographically defined general population. *Neurology* 2010; **75**(14): 1249–55.

Further reading

Knopman DS, Petersen RC, Cha RH, Edland SD, Rocca WA. Incidence and causes of nondegenerative nonvascular dementia: a population-based study. *Arch Neurol* 2006; **63**(2): 218–21.

Ridha B, Josephs KA. Young-onset dementia: a practical approach to diagnosis. *Neurologist* 2006; **12**(1): 2–13.

Rossor MN, Fox NC, Mummery CJ, Schott JM, Warren JD. The diagnosis of young-onset dementia. *Lancet Neurol* 2010; **9**(8): 793–806.

Sampson EL, Warren JD, Rossor MN. Young onset dementia. *Postgrad Med J* 2004; **80**(941): 125–39.

Shinagawa S, Ikeda M, Toyota Y, et al. Frequency and clinical characteristics of early-onset dementia in consecutive patients in a memory clinic. *Dement Geriatr Cogn Disord* 2007; **24**(1): 42–7.

Snowden JS, Thompson JC, Stopford CL, et al. The clinical diagnosis of early-onset dementias: diagnostic accuracy and clinicopathological relationships. *Brain* 2011; **134**(Pt 9): 2478–92.

Warren JD, Schott JM, Fox NC, et al. Brain biopsy in dementia. *Brain* 2005; **128**(Pt 9): 2016–25.

Wicklund MR, Mokri B, Drubach DA, Boeve BF, Parisi JE, Josephs KA. Frontotemporal brain sagging syndrome: an SIH-like presentation mimicking FTD. *Neurology* 2011; **76**(16): 1377–82.

4

An Approach to the Problem of Normal Pressure Hydrocephalus

Norman Relkin

Department of Neurology and Neuroscience, Weill Medical College of Cornell University, USA

Introduction

Hakim and Adams described the classic symptom triad of shuffling gait, urinary incontinence, and dementia in 1965 and are credited with the identification of normal pressure hydrocephalus (NPH) as a surgically treatable neurological condition[1]. NPH is now widely recognized as a potentially reversible cause of physical disability and cognitive impairment in the elderly.

Demographics

Normal pressure hydrocephalus most commonly affects persons over 50 years of age and may occur alone or in combination with age-related disorders such as Alzheimer's, Lewy body, and Parkinson's disease. NPH is found in roughly equal numbers of males and females. Familial association has been anecdotally reported but is only rarely encountered in practice. The precise incidence and prevalence of NPH have not been rigorously determined. A Norwegian study in over 20,000 subjects estimated incidence of NPH at 5.5 per 100,000 population and prevalence at 21.9 per 100,000 population[2].

Classification of normal pressure hydrocephalus

Normal pressure hydrocephalus is one of many different forms of hydrocephalus and has several distinguishing features.

Normal pressure hydrocephalus is:

- a chronic form of hydrocephalus in adults
- a "communicating" form of hydrocephalus in which ventricular enlargement occurs in the absence of a macroscopic obstruction to the flow of cerebrospinal fluid (CSF). The term "communicating" refers to the free flow of CSF between the ventricular chambers and the other conduits for CSF flow
- associated with near normal static intracranial pressure (ICP). The ICP in NPH patients may be as low as 70 mmH$_2$O or as high as 230 mmH$_2$O. Higher ICP usually indicates another process such as an intracranial mass or an obstructive form of hydrocephalus
- associated with disturbances of gait and balance, control of urination and/or impairment of cognition. These three domains comprise the "classic triad" of NPH
- either "idiopathic" (no identifiable antecedent) or "secondary" to conditions such as intracranial hemorrhage, meningitis or head trauma.

Normal pressure hydrocephalus is not:

- an acute disorder. In most cases, acute hydrocephalus is due to macroscopic obstructions to CSF flow by space-occupying lesions
- brain atrophy. Shrinkage of the brain, which occurs in aging as well as degenerative diseases,

Dementia, First Edition. Edited by Joseph F. Quinn.

causes ventricular enlargement that is sometimes called "hydrocephalus *ex vacuo*." In practice, differentiating NPH from *ex vacuo* enlargement of the ventricles can be challenging (see Neuroimaging section below)

- a congenital or childhood form of hydrocephalus, although some possible links to childhood forms have been hypothesized (see Pathophysiology section below)
- the consequence of aqueductal stenosis (AS). AS can closely resemble NPH but differs in cause and treatment. In AS, congenital or acquired narrowing of the aqueduct of Silvius leads to ventricular enlargement and symptoms quite similar to NPH. Stenosis of the aqueduct can be identified on a midsagittal magnetic resonance imaging (MRI) scan, particularly high-resolution anatomical sequences such as constructive interference in steady state (CISS), and by flow-sensitive MRI techniques that document diminished CSF flow rates.

Pathophysiology

The causes of NPH are incompletely understood. Possible links between NPH and certain abnormalities of early childhood have been noted.

- Head circumference is often (but not always) increased in patients with NPH. According to the so-called "two hit" hypothesis of NPH, benign congenital external hydrocephalus (increased CSF compartment external to the brain) combined with the development of deep white matter ischemia later in life may lead to NPH in older adults[3]. Since skull size becomes fixed after the fontanelles close in early childhood, untreated external hydrocephalus in childhood could provide an explanation why head circumference is increased in a significant subset of patients with NPH[3].

☆ TIPS AND TRICKS

Head circumference above the 90th percentile for age and height is associated with a three-fold increased risk of adult hydrocephalus[4].

- Another NPH-like syndrome related to childhood hydrocephalus is called "long-standing overt ventriculomegaly in adults (LOVA)[5]." LOVA is thought to begin with childhood hydrocephalus that is initially compensated but progresses later in life to cause symptoms. Associated findings include an enlarged head circumference and in some cases an empty sella turcica.

Several lines of evidence indicate that CSF pulsatility is disturbed in NPH. High CSF pulse pressures (despite normal or near normal static ICP) could physically distort the ventricles and alter the normal pathways for the clearance of cerebrospinal fluid. CSF is produced intraventricularly by arterial pulsations in the choroid plexus. It then circulates down through the cerebrospinal cavity before returning to the superior sagittal sinus (SSS) where it is cleared via absorption by arachnoid villi. In NPH, clearance through the SSS may be impeded as a result of compression of its tributary veins during the cardiac cycle[6]. It has been noted that some patients with NPH have enlarged subarachnoid spaces (SAS) toward the ventral and middle portions of the brain but reduced spaces around the superior sagittal sinus (see Neuroimaging section, below). This is thought to indicate an altered pathway of CSF circulation in NPH in which increased bulk reflux of CSF occurs into ventricles during diastole, fostering reverse transependymal CSF flow and clearance through lateral venous sinuses.

⟐ SCIENCE REVISITED

The Monro–Kelli Doctrine, hyperdynamic CSF flow and venous pulsations in NPH
The adult skull is a closed, non-distensible space. Each time the heart beats, arterial blood flows into the cranial cavity under pressure. According to the Monro–Kelli Doctrine, the volume of the arterial inflow must be equal to the volume of CSF and venous blood that leaves the cranial cavity. Net input must equal net output.

Normally, the brain is compliant enough that the energy of each cardiac pulsation is partially transferred to brain tissue, resulting in outward radial expansion of the ventricles. In NPH, the ventricles become maximally enlarged. As a result, most of the energy of

> arterial pulsation is transferred to the CSF and venous system. This can result in rapid "hyperdynamic" CSF flow through the aqueduct of Silvius, third ventricle and fourth ventricle that can be detected by phase contrast MRI, as well as pulsatile venous flow.

It is not entirely known how disturbances in the CSF compartment translate into brain dysfunction and the clinical symptoms in NPH. Static ICP is inadequately elevated in NPH to cause cerebral dysfunction in itself. However, ventricular distension and widened dynamic CSF pulse pressures may be sufficient to compress capacitance vessels in the brain, reducing their availability to increase cerebral perfusion during periods of peak demand. Reduced cortical cerebral blood flow can occur in NPH, but overall brain perfusion is not universally compromised nor is it consistently improved after treatment. Small vessel ischemic cerebrovascular disease is nevertheless linked to progression of NPH. As the burden of cerebrovascular disease increases, NPH generally becomes more refractory to treatment. In chronically untreated cases, small vessel infarction occurs throughout the periventricular region, giving rise to a condition that is virtually indistinguishable from Binswanger's disease.

Ventricular expansion, transependymal fluid movement and age-associated reductions in cerebral compliance may make the brain more susceptible to the repeated impact of the CSF pulsations. Physical distortion of neurons and their periventricular processes caused by ventricular enlargement has been hypothesized to delay or disrupt neuronal transmission in NPH.

Pathological studies have failed to identify lesions at the gross or molecular levels that are universally diagnostic of NPH or unequivocally explain its etiology Not surprisingly, the most consistent finding in NPH patients at autopsy is simply enlargement of the cerebral ventricles.

Symptoms

Normal pressure hydrocephalus is associated with gait ataxia, urinary incontinence, and dementia. Symptoms fall on a continuum from very mild to quite severe and are not limited to those of the classic triad. Symptoms are stage dependent, and may be minimal early in the disease and/or confined to just one or two domains of the triad. It is important for clinicians to become familiar with the full spectrum of presentations and stages of NPH.

Gait and balance

Impairments of walking and balance are the most readily observed symptoms of NPH and the most reliably reversed by treatment.

- The characteristic gait disturbance in NPH is variably described as "magnetic," "shuffling" or glue-footed."
- Patients with NPH typically show a reduced foot–floor clearance and a widened base, walking in short steps with their toes pointed outward. The number of steps required to cover a given distance is often increased as a result.
- There is reduced counterrotation of the hips and shoulders while walking. Accelerometer studies show an increased tendency to sway while walking as well as standing in place.
- Tandem gait is frequently disturbed, although this is observed in many elderly patients without NPH.
- It often takes symptomatic NPH patients longer than normal to rise from a chair and to walk a short distance.
- Patients with NPH frequently fall backward (retropulse) either spontaneously or as a consequence of being pulled backwards on the "Pull Test."
- Turning in place may require multiple small steps, so-called "*en bloc*" turning.
- NPH patients often fall directly forward or backward when bending or on uneven terrain, but can fall in any direction.
- There may be a prolonged latency when starting ambulation or stopping, a symptom overlapping that of idiopathic Parkinson's disease (PD). Parkinsonism may be present in NPH patients either as a co-morbid illness or as a consequence of NPH itself. Parkinsonism secondary to NPH tends to be less responsive to treatment with dopamine precursors or agonists than in uncomplicated PD.

A timed walking test over a set distance is an inexpensive and sensitive method for identifying and following the gait disturbances in NPH. Standardized clinical gait assessment is useful for rating the full range of associated gait and balance disturbances.

Control of urination

The most common urinary symptoms in NPH are frequency, urgency, and nocturia. These early symptoms may progress to urinary incontinence as the disease progresses. In most cases, incontinence is confined to micturition but in advanced stages defecation may be involved as well. NPH patients are initially aware of their urinary symptoms and embarrassed when incontinence develops. With progression of the disease and particularly with advancing dementia, they may develop indifference to incontinence.

Asking subjects or spouses to keep a bladder diary indicating frequency/urgency of urination and incidents of incontinence can provide useful diagnostic information. Urological evaluation is recommended to rule out other causes of urinary dysfunction. Urodynamic studies in NPH patients tend to show a neurogenic-type pattern and may reveal an increased postvoid residual. Persons with untreated NPH may be at increased risk of urinary tract infections (UTI) owing to incomplete voiding. Those with recurrent UTIs may benefit from antimicrobial prophylaxis.

Cognition

The profile of cognitive impairments in NPH is typically "subcortical" with frontally weighted deficits and relative sparing of language function. Not infrequently, NPH occurs in combination with diseases such as Alzheimer's which may add elements of cortical, limbic, and paralimbic disturbances to the profile of cognitive dysfunction. Cognitive impairment in NPH often manifests as a disturbance of executive function, with difficulties carrying out multistep tasks, multitasking, formulating abstractions, and dividing attention. Memory loss is often secondary to impaired information retrieval. Recognition memory is relatively preserved as evidenced by performance improving with cues or multiple choice. This contrasts with Alzheimer's disease in which the information is rapidly lost from memory and may neither be recalled or recognized. Language ability usually remains intact, although phonemic (letter) fluency and confrontational naming are decreased in conjunction with frontal systems deficits. Ideomotor praxis may be preserved

but some patients with NPH have difficulty transitioning from a standing to a recumbent position such as on an examining table.

Screening tests such as the Folstein Mini Mental State Examination may not be sufficiently sensitive to detect subtle frontal systems deficits in NPH. Timed performance-based tasks and tasks with frontal weightings are recommended to assess impairments in suspected cases of NPH. Tests such as Trails B and the Symbol-Digit Test tend to be sensitive to NPH-related deficits as well as to improvement with treatment. Certain tests of upper extremity function (maze drawing and serial dotting) have recently been found sensitive to impairments in NPH and are responsive to CSF drainage[7]. Neuropsychological testing can be useful in documenting subtle cognitive dysfunction in mild stages of NPH and for tracking response to treatment.

Other findings

A variety of psychiatric disturbances ranging from psychosis and agitation to depression and anxiety disorders have been reported in association with NPH, either as exacerbation of preexisting conditions or arising de novo. In some cases, psychiatric symptoms are responsive to treatment of hydrocephalus. Recent onset of hypertension has been reported in an unexpected fraction of patients with newly diagnosed NPH, leading to the speculation of a possible causal relationship. Decreased hearing and frank deafness have been rarely associated with NPH, but primarily in the aftermath of shunt placement rather than as presenting symptoms. The same is true of epilepsy, which may occur in as many as 10% of shunted NH patients.

Diagnostic criteria

International consensus criteria for the diagnosis of idiopathic NPH were published in 2005[8]. These evidence-based guidelines divide NPH into probable and possible subcategories to reflect the level of certainty about the diagnosis. The guidelines also identify "shunt-responsive NPH" as the subset of cases that have a positive outcome from treatment. The criteria for probable and possible INPH are listed in Box 4.1.

Differential diagnosis

The symptoms of NPH overlap those of several conditions that are common in elderly individuals. Alzheimer's disease, Parkinson's disease and other

Box 4.1 International consensus criteria for idiopathic normal pressure hydrocephalus

Probable idiopathic NPH

The diagnosis of probable idiopathic NPH is based on clinical history, brain imaging, physical findings, and physiological criteria

I. History

Reported symptoms should be corroborated by an informant familiar with the patient's premorbid and current condition, and must include:

a. Insidious onset (versus acute)
b. Origin after age 40 years
c. A minimum duration of at least 3–6 months
d. No evidence of an antecedent event such as head trauma, intracerebral hemorrhage, meningitis, or other known causes of secondary hydrocephalus
e. Progression over time
f. No other neurological, psychiatric, or general medical conditions that are sufficient to explain the presenting symptoms

II. Brain imaging

A brain imaging study (CT or MRI) performed after onset of symptoms must show evidence of:

a. Ventricular enlargement not entirely attributable to cerebral atrophy or congenital enlargement (Evans Index >0.3 or comparable measure)
b. No macroscopic obstruction to CSF flow
c. At least one of the following supportive features:
    1. Enlargement of the temporal horns of the lateral ventricles not entirely attributable to hippocampus atrophy
    2. Callosal angle of 40° or more
    3. Evidence of altered brain water content, including periventricular signal changes on CT and MRI not attributable to microvascular ischemic changes or demyelination
    4. An aqueductal or fourth ventricular flow void on MRI

Other brain imaging findings may be supportive of an idiopathic NPH diagnosis but are not required for a probable designation:

a. A brain imaging study performed before onset of symptoms showing smaller ventricular size or without evidence of hydrocephalus
b. Radionuclide cisternogram showing delayed clearance of radiotracer over the cerebral convexities after 48–72 h
c. Cine MRI study or other technique showing increased ventricular flow rate
d. A SPECT-acetazolamide challenge showing decreased periventricular perfusion that is not altered by acetazolamide

III. Clinical

Findings of gait/balance disturbance must be present, plus at least one other area of impairment in cognition, urinary symptoms, or both

With respect to gait/balance, at least two of the following should be present and not be entirely attributable to other conditions:

a. Decreased step height
b. Decreased step length
c. Decreased cadence (speed of walking)
d. Increased trunk sway during walking
e. Widened standing base
f. Toes turned outward on walking
g. Retropulsion (spontaneous or provoked)
h. *En bloc* turning (turning requiring three or more steps for 180°)
i. Impaired walking balance, as evidenced by two or more corrections out of eight steps on tandem gait testing

With respect to cognition, there must be documented impairment (adjusted for age and educational attainment) and/or decrease in performance on a cognitive screening instrument (such as the Minimental State Examination), or evidence of at least two of the following on examination that is not fully attributable to other conditions:

a. Psychomotor slowing (increased response latency)
b. Decreased fine motor speed
c. Decreased fine motor accuracy
d. Difficulty dividing or maintaining attention
e. Impaired recall, especially for recent events
f. Executive dysfunction, such as impairment in multistep procedures, working memory, formulation of abstractions/similarities, insight
g. Behavioral or personality changes

To document symptoms in the domain of urinary continence, one of the following should be present:

a. Episodic or persistent urinary incontinence not attributable to primary urological disorders
b. Persistent urinary incontinence
c. Urinary and fecal incontinence

Or any two of the following should be present:

a. Urinary urgency as defined by frequent perception of a pressing need to void
b. Urinary frequency as defined by more than six voiding episodes in an average 12-h period despite normal fluid intake
c. Nocturia as defined by the need to urinate more than two times in an average night

IV. Physiological

CSF opening pressure in the range of 5–18 mm Hg (or 70–245 mmH$_2$O) as determined by a lumbar puncture or a comparable procedure. Appropriately measured pressures that are significantly higher or lower than this range are not consistent with a probable NPH diagnosis

Possible idiopathic NPH

A diagnosis of possible idiopathic NPH is based on historical, brain imaging, and clinical and physiological criteria

I. History

Reported symptoms may:

a. Have a subacute or indeterminate mode of onset
b. Begin at any age after childhood
c. May have less than 3 months or indeterminate duration
d. May follow events such as mild head trauma, remote history of intracerebral hemorrhage, or childhood and adolescent meningitis or other conditions that in the judgment of the clinician are not likely to be causally related
e. Co-exist with other neurological, psychiatric, or general medical disorders but in the judgment of the clinician not be entirely attributable to these conditions
f. Be non-progressive or not clearly progressive

II. Brain imaging

Ventricular enlargement consistent with hydrocephalus but associated with either of the following:

a. Evidence of cerebral atrophy of sufficient severity to potentially explain ventricular size
b. Structural lesions that may influence ventricular size

III. Clinical

Symptoms of either:

a. Incontinence and/or cognitive impairment in the absence of an observable gait or balance disturbance
b. Gait disturbance or dementia alone

IV. Physiological

Opening pressure measurement not available or pressure outside the range required for probable idiopathic NPH

Unlikely idiopathic NPH

1. No evidence of ventriculomegaly
2. Signs of increased intracranial pressure such as papilledema
3. No component of the clinical triad of idiopathic NPH is present
4. Symptoms explained by other causes (e.g. spinal stenosis)

Reproduced from Relkin et al[8]. with permission from Lippincott Williams and Wilkins.

neurodegenerative conditions can manifest similar symptoms and may occur coincidentally with NPH. Spinal stenosis, arthritic conditions, and orthopedic disorders can cause gait and balance disturbances resembling those of NPH. Prostatic enlargement and a number of other urological conditions can give rise to the urgency, frequency, and incontinence that are also associated with NPH. Differential diagnosis of NPH therefore requires careful exclusion of other conditions, while appreciating that some cases of NPH occur in the setting of co-morbidities. The challenge when such conditions are found becomes determination of the extent to which symptoms are attributable to NPH versus the co-morbidities.

Neuroimaging

A brain imaging study is necessary to identify ventricular enlargement in NPH but diagnosis also requires documentation of appropriate clinical findings. X-ray computed tomography (CT) or nuclear medicine scans such as cisternography can be used for this purpose, but MRI is the preferred modality for evaluating NPH. The use of MRI is limited by contraindications such as pacemakers, metallic implants, and claustrophobia, as well as in some venues by cost and availability. A T1-weighted or other MRI pulse sequence that highlights ventricular and cortical anatomy can readily be used for this purpose.

Since ventricular enlargement also occurs in aging and neurodegenerative diseases, evaluation of possible NPH requires making a determination of whether the enlargement of the ventricles is disproportionate to cerebral atrophy (see Figure 4.1). This is currently accomplished by visual inspection of brain images to identify widened sulcal markings as proxy measures of brain atrophy. This method is highly subjective and may soon be supplanted by quantitative MRI volumetric techniques that provide more accurate measures of cortical atrophy. Advances in MRI methods and other imaging techniques are likely to contribute to improved differential diagnosis of NPH in the future.

> ⭐ **TIPS AND TRICKS**
>
> **Measuring ventricular enlargement**
> The Evans Index is a measure of ventricular size calculated from the ratio of the diameter of the anterior horn of the lateral ventricle to the skull's widest diameter. An Evans Index of 0.3 or greater is required for an NPH diagnosis but this may also be found in patients with ventricular enlargement from other causes.

Imaging can also be useful for verifying whether there is any obstruction to CSF flow. In cases with past spinal surgery or myelopathic symptoms, imaging of the spine is recommended. Inspection of a midline sagittal T1-weighted image is recommended for examining the patency of the cerebral aqueduct and fourth ventricle. In equivocal cases, a phase contrast CSF flow study can provide useful information about CSF movement. Aqueductal flow rates are low or undetectable in aqueductal stenosis, while in NPH normal or increased (hyperdynamic) flow is observed. High-speed imaging techniques

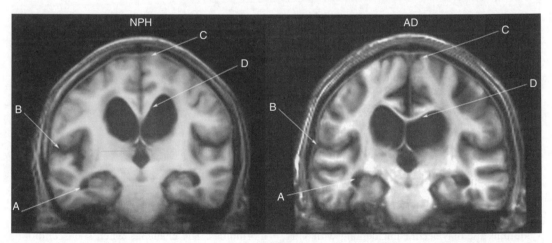

Figure 4.1 Coronal T1-weighted MRI images comparing patient with NPH (*left*) to patient with Alzheimer's disease (*right*). Arrow A: Temporal horns are enlarged in both conditions. In NPH this is due to ventricular enlargement whereas in AD this is attributable to mesial temporal atrophy. Arrow B: Subarachnoid space is expanded in both conditions, but in NPH there is often accentuated involvement of the ventral sulci and fissures, whereas in AD the distribution of sulcal widening is more uniform. Arrow C: The sulci in the high parietal convexity appear tightened in NPH and closely opposed to the sagittal sinus. Arrow D: The callosal angle is 90° or less in NPH owing to upward bowing of the roof of the lateral ventricles, while in AD it is typically more obtuse.

such as CISS and fast imaging employing steady state acquisition (FIESTA) MRI sequences can be useful for identifying small obstructions. Hyperdynamic flow can sometimes be identified as a fourth ventricular flow void on proton density images or non-water suppressed echo planar images.

Other structural findings associated with NPH that can be identified on CT scans or MRIs include enlargement of the temporal horns of the lateral ventricles not attributable to hippocampal atrophy, upward doming of the roof of the body of lateral ventricles, enlargement of the Sylvian fissure and compression of the paramedian sulci of the frontoparietal region near the cranial convexity (see Figure 4.1, arrow C).

Prognosis

Some generalizations can be made about the likelihood of a positive response to shunt treatment based on demographic and medical history, and additional prognostication can be made on the basis of clinical tests.

- Prognosis for a positive response to neurosurgical treatment in NPH is better for patients age 75 years or less, with duration of symptoms less than 2 years and a lack of serious medical co-morbidities. A less favorable prognosis is associated with atypical presentations, advanced dementia, long-standing symptoms, confluent subcortical cerebrovascular changes, and concomitant anticoagulation therapy.
- Several tests have been developed to estimate the likelihood that a person with NPH will respond positively to a shunt. These techniques include high-volume (30–50 cc) lumbar puncture "tap tests," 24–72-h external lumbar or ventricular catheter drainage, CSF dynamics studies, MRI CSF flow measurements, B-wave monitoring and radionuclide cisternography and others. While positive results on these tests can indicate a more favorable prognosis for shunt response, negative outcomes do not preclude benefit from a shunt. For that reason, these tests tend to be used selectively in cases in which the decision about whether or not to proceed to shunt must be balanced against increased risks. The likelihood of shunt responsiveness can be determined with up to 90% specificity when prognostic tests are positive[9].

✋ CAUTION

Look before you tap!

- Performing a high-volume lumbar puncture (LP) in the presence of an obstruction to CSF flow can result in worsening of symptoms or even brain herniation and death.
- Obstruction to the flow of CSF can occur in the absence of papilledema or other signs of increased intracranial pressure.
- A CT scan or MRI should be carried out before performing an LP or other drainage procedure. *The presence of a complete obstruction to CSF flow should be considered a contraindication to performing LP or other drainage procedures below the level of the obstruction.*

Treatment

A distinctive feature of NPH is that its symptoms can be rapidly reversed by procedures that divert CSF out of the central nervous system. Temporary improvements can occur after LP, external lumbar drainage (ELD), and ventriculostomy. Lasting reversal of symptoms follows neurosurgical implantation of a ventricular shunt. Shunt placement is standard of care for NPH and fosters excellent recovery in well-selected patients.

Shunts are permanent implanted devices that serve as an alternative physical conduit for the outflow of CSF from the central nervous system. Shunts have many different designs and configurations, and are reviewed elsewhere[10]. The most basic configuration is a tube running from the cerebral ventricles to another location in the body in which drainage occurs by gravity. In most cases, however, a shunt valve is introduced between the two ends to control the rate and volume of drainage of CSF as the position of the head relative to the rest of the body changes. The most common type of shunt in use today is a differential pressure valve that opens when a certain pressure difference exists between the ventricular side of the shunt and its distal end, which is most often placed intraabdominally. The shunt valve may be supplemented by an antisyphon device that prevents the valve from remaining open when gravity induces a rapid flow (syphon) effect.

Until the 1990s, most shunt valves had fixed opening pressures (low, medium, and high). An important innovation that changed the management of NPH was the advent of programmable valves that can be non-invasively adjusted postoperatively. Current programmable valves can be adjusted by magnetic or electromagnetic programming devices and can be set non-invasively to a wide range of opening pressures. This provides an opportunity to optimize the shunt function in individual cases and a way to adjust the extent of drainage. The settings of a programmable shunt can be interrogated by various means that are valve dependent, including magnetic compass devices, acoustic devices, and x-rays. The value of programmable shunts relative to reduction of shunt morbidity compared to fixed pressure shunts has not been conclusively established, but they have given NPH patients and their physicians greater latitude to manage symptoms that would otherwise require repeated surgery.

While shunts can provide relief to well-chosen surgical candidates that persists for several years, the outcome of shunt placement is not uniformly positive. Shunts fail to provide improvement in some cases and are associated with operative and postoperative morbidity rates ranging from 10% to 80% in different case series. Complications such as subdural hematomas, infections, and shunt blockage take a devastating toll on frail, elderly NPH patients and dramatically increase the costs of NPH care. Maximizing successful treatment of NPH requires accurate diagnosis and skillful clinical management by specifically trained healthcare professionals.

Long-standing overt ventriculomegaly in adults (LOVA) and AS may be treatable by endoscopic third ventriculostomy (ETV), a procedure that creates an alternative conduit for CSF flow through the floor of the third ventricle. ETV may be associated with lower morbidity than shunts typically used to treat NPH but does not reverse symptoms in all cases.

Non-surgical aspects of management are also extremely important for the care of patients with NPH. In both the presurgical and postsurgical periods, vulnerability to falling is increased and appropriate measures should be taken to reduce fall risk. This can be promoted by prescription of a cane, walker or, when appropriate, a wheelchair. Modifications to the household should be considered for safety purposes, including but not limited to installation of grab bars in the bathroom and handrails on ramps and stairwells. Suitable candidates should be referred for physical therapy. A program of scheduled toileting may help those prone to UTIs or daytime incontinence, and prescription of prophylaxis against UTIs should be considered in some cases. Medications such as cholinesterase inhibitors that are approved to treat Alzheimer's disease and dementia in Parkinson's disease have not been formally evaluated in NPH but may have adjunct therapeutic value in some patients. The same may be said about dopamine precursors such as levodopa. Focal or generalized seizure may emerge after shunt surgery and should be addressed with antiepileptic medication if recurrent. Depression and other behavioral disturbances also occur in the NPH population and may require medication and/or psychotherapy. In patients with advanced symptoms or who are not candidates for surgery, a home health aide or even institutionalization may become necessary. This is particularly the case for individuals who live alone or are more physically frail or severely demented.

There are no established pharmacological treatments for NPH. Anecdotal evidence has been forwarded for the use of low-dose acetazolamide (250–500 mg/day) either alone or in combination with serial LPs. Additional studies are needed to improve surgical management of NPH as well as increasing the options for non-surgical treatment.

Conclusion

Normal pressure hydrocephalus is a chronic form of adult hydrocephalus that is treatable and sometimes reversible. Idiopathic and secondary forms exist and the pathophysiology is incompletely understood.

Diagnosis of NPH requires evidence of ventricular enlargement disproportionate to cerebral atrophy on a brain imaging study and impairment in gait, balance, continence, and/or cognition. MRI or another brain imaging study is required. Clinical assessment must include appropriate history and physical examination.

The classic triad of gait ataxia, incontinence, and dementia is sometimes but not always present in NPH patients and can occur in other disorders. Impairments may be mild and/or in a single domain.

Symptoms of NPH may overlap those of Parkinson's disease, Alzheimer's disease and other disorders even when NPH occurs in isolation.

The cognitive profile of NPH is typically "subcortical" with predominant frontally weighted deficits. Not infrequently, NPH occurs in combination with diseases such as Alzheimer's which may add elements of cortical, limbic, and paralimbic disturbances to the cognitive profile.

Gait disturbance tends to be the most responsive to treatment. Balance, control of urination, and cognition follow respectively in terms of likelihood and time to improvement.

Invasive examinations such as lumbar drainage, infusion tests, and ICP monitoring may add to diagnostic and prognostic certainty but are not required in every case.

Neurosurgical placement of a shunt that diverts CSF away from the brain in a controlled fashion is the current treatment of choice for NPH. Ventriculoperitoneal shunt is the most common configuration and shunt valves may be fixed or adjustable pressure types. Success rates can be as high as 90% but vary across centers. Endoscopic third ventriculostomy, devices to alter CSF pulsatility, and medications are under study but are not of proven value in NPH.

Although mortality attributable to shunt surgery is generally low, postoperative morbidity from shunts is 10–15% or higher. Subdural hematomas and effusions are common complications. Seizures, infections, and shunt failures are among other serious adverse consequences. Factors such as advanced age, multiple medical co-morbidities, extreme frailty, anticoagulation, and severe dementia increase the risk of adverse outcomes from shunt surgery.

Accurate diagnosis, skilled surgical intervention, and careful long-term management are required to minimize morbidity and treat NPH successfully.

References

[1] Hakim S, Adams RD. The special clinical problem of symptomatic hydrocephalus with normal cerebrospinal fluid pressure. Observations on cerebrospinal fluid hydrodynamics. *J Neurol Sci* 1965; **2**(4): 307–27.

[2] Brean A, Eide PK. Prevalence of probable idiopathic normal pressure hydrocephalus in a Norwegian population. *Acta Neurol Scand* 2008; **118**(1): 48–53.

[3] Bradley W, Bahl G, Alksne J. Idiopathic normal pressure hydrocephalus may be a "two hit" disease: benign external hydrocephalus in infancy followed by deep white matter ischemia in late adulthood. *J Mag Res Imaging* 2006; **24**(4): 747–55.

[4] Krefft T, Graff-Radford N, Lucas J, Mortimer J. Normal pressure hydrocephalus and large head size. *Alzheimer Dis Assoc Disord* 2004; **18**(1): 35–7.

[5] Kiefer M, Eymann R, Steudel W. I LOVA hydrocephalus – a new entity of chronic hydrocephalus. *Der Nervenarzt* 2002; **73**(10): 972–81.

[6] Bateman G. The pathophysiology of idiopathic normal pressure hydrocephalus: cerebral ischemia or altered venous hemodynamics. *Am J Neuroradiol* 2008; **29**:198–203.

[7] Tsakanikas D, Katzen H, Ravdin L, Relkin N. Upper extremity motor measures of tap test response in normal pressure hydrocephalus. *Clin Neurol Neurosurg* 2009; **111**(9): 752–7.

[8] Relkin N, Marmarou A, Klinge P, Bergsneider M, Black P. Diagnosing idiopathic normal-pressure hydrocephalus. *Neurosurgery* 2005; **57**(3): S2-4–S2-16.

[9] Marmarou A, Bergsneider, M, Klinge P, Relkin N, Black P. The value of supplemental prognostic tests for the preoperative assessment of idiopathic normal-pressure hydrocephalus. *J Neurosurg* 2005; **57**(3): S17–S28.

[10] Bergsneider M, Black PM, Klinge P, Marmarou A, Relkin N. Surgical management of idiopathic normal-pressure hydrocephalus. *Neurosurg Online* 2005; **57**(Suppl. 3): S29–39.

5

Depression: Cause or Complication of Cognitive Decline?

David Mansoor, Sahana Misra and Linda Ganzini

Portland Veterans Affairs Medical Center, Oregon Health and Science University, USA

Introduction

Depression may be a risk factor, prodrome, correlate or outcome of dementia. This chapter will provide the reader with a general understanding of geriatric depression and the relationship between depression and cognitive impairment, and a clinical approach to diagnosis and treatment of depression in the elderly, focusing on those with cognitive impairment.

CASE

Mr S is a 72-year-old man who told his primary care provider that he had depressed and low mood, poor sleep with the inability to sleep past 4.00 am, reduced appetite, and loss of interest in hobbies, all over the past 3 months. He was concerned that he had become more "forgetful." He scored 11 out of 15 on the Geriatric Depression Scale (GDS), indicating severe depression. He scored 23 out of 30 on the Saint Louis University Mental Status Examination (SLUMS) indicating mild cognitive impairment; on cognitive testing, however, he seemed to give up easily and answered many questions with "I'm not sure." Mr S had experienced a period of depression in his early 20s, which resolved without treatment after about 6 months. His other medical problems included hypertension, hyperlipidemia, and type 2 diabetes mellitus.

His primary care provider diagnosed him as having a major depressive disorder and started the selective serotonin reuptake inhibitor (SSRI) sertraline. At an appointment 3 months later Mr S reported that his mood was improved and he had renewed interest in his hobbies. On the 15-point GDS his score was 3, indicating very few depression symptoms, and his SLUMS improved to 29 out of 30.

Current understanding of geriatric depression and the relationship between depression and cognitive impairment

The term depression is used both colloquially and medically, but in both instances indicates feeling blue, sad or unhappy. Medically the term is most often synonymous with major depressive disorder, a psychiatric illness characterized by persistent low mood and/or loss of pleasure and interest in normally enjoyable activities accompanied by changes in sleep and appetite, impaired concentration or difficulty with decision making, low energy, agitated or lethargic motor activity, feelings of worthlessness or inappropriate guilt, and thoughts of dying (see Box 5.1). These symptoms must be present for at least 2 weeks, and must negatively influence functioning or create disruption in the patient's life. We will use the terms depression and major depressive disorder interchangeably. Researchers use the term

Dementia, First Edition. Edited by Joseph F. Quinn.

> ### Box 5.1 DSM-IV-TR diagnostic criteria for major depressive disorder
>
> Depressed mood
> Anhedonia (loss of interest or pleasure in
>   activities)
> Changes in weight or appetite
> Changes in sleep (insomnia or hypersomnia)
> Psychomotor agitation or retardation
> Low energy
> Feelings of worthlessness or guilt
> Poor concentration or difficulty making
>   decisions
> Recurrent suicidal ideation or thoughts of death
>
> (five or more symptoms present for a 2-week
> period, including either depressed mood or
> anhedonia)

subsyndromal depression to refer to mood disorders that do not meet full diagnostic criteria for major depressive disorder, either because the symptoms are present for less than 2 weeks or the patient experiences fewer depression symptoms. Yet patients with this seemingly less severe form of depression have negative outcomes similar to major depressive disorder including greater medical co-morbidity, diminished social activity, functional decline, and higher utilization of healthcare services. They are also at risk for developing major depressive disorder and suicidal ideation.

Depression is neither a normal nor expected development in old age. The prevalence of major depressive disorder in community-dwelling persons over the age of 65 is only 1%, less than that for middle-aged adults. However, the prevalence increases as the burden of age-related medical illness and functional impairments increases. For example, one study estimated the prevalence of major depression in elderly hospitalized patients to be 11.5%, and 13.5% in those who required home healthcare. Some depressive symptoms are ubiquitous in patients with Alzheimer's disease, occurring in up to 87% of patients; prevalence estimates of major depression vary, though most reports estimate the prevalence to be 20–25%. In a study of long-term care residents, the incidence of major depressive disorder among those with Alzheimer's

disease was estimated at 6% over 1 year. Depression also complicates the course of less commonly occurring dementias, including, for example, vascular dementia, Parkinson's disease dementia, and dementia due to Huntington's disease.

Depression develops most commonly in the early and middle stages of Alzheimer's disease. Aalten and co-investigators followed 199 patients with dementia, mostly Alzheimer's disease, for 2 years and found that depression became less prevalent and less severe with disease progression while apathy and aberrant motor behavior, such as pacing, fidgeting, and inability to sit still, increased. Depression in patients with dementia is associated with a higher prevalence of other problematic behaviors, such as wandering and verbal agitation.

> **EVIDENCE AT A GLANCE**
>
> Depression becomes less prevalent and less severe with progression of dementia, while apathy and increased motor activity such as wandering and restlessness tend to increase.

The frequent co-occurrence of depression and dementia was first recognized in the 1880s, when the French psychiatrist Albert Mairet described melancholic depression, a disorder in which both poor mood and cognitive impairment were prominent. In 1952, the term "pseudodementia" was used by John Madden to describe older patients whose cognitive impairment developed and remitted with successful treatment of depression. Other geropsychiatrists have referred to this clinical presentation as "dementia syndrome of depression" and "depression related to cognitive dysfunction." Despite decades of recognition and interest, researchers still do not agree on the clinical criteria for pseudodementia, yet describe similar characteristics.

In general, patients with pseudodementia complain of global memory decline, with emphasis on disability and subjective distress. They frequently exhibit slowed physical movement, anxiety, and neurovegetative symptoms of depression such as disrupted sleep, changes in appetite, and poor concentration. Their thoughts are marked by a sense of guilt and hopelessness that they will not improve or that any aspect of the future will be pleasurable. Scores on cognitive testing can be lower than expected for their level of function as a result of poor effort, for example, answering, "I don't know" to even the simplest tests of cognition. In contrast to Alzheimer's disease, sustained attention and motor speed are more impaired than delayed recall and object naming, and patients are typically capable of retaining information once learned.

> ### ★ TIPS AND TRICKS
>
> Patients with pseudodementia often complain of memory impairment and show poor effort on cognitive examination. In these patients cognitive impairment may initially improve with depression treatment, but most will ultimately develop Alzheimer's disease.

Pseudodementia is not always a benign condition. Several types of studies support the theory that a large subset of patients with pseudodementia in fact have early Alzheimer's disease. For example, in a study employing functional neuroimaging, Cho and co-authors showed decreased cerebral blood flow in the temporoparietal region in patients with pseudodementia, similar to that of the Alzheimer's disease comparators and different from the depressed study participants. Autopsy studies reveal that structural brain changes in patients with pseudodementia and Alzheimer's dementia are similar. Prospective studies of patients with pseudodementia concur that cognition improves after depression treatment, yet up to 89% of patients subsequently develop dementia, usually Alzheimer's dementia. Overall, these studies add strength to the finding that pseudodementia presages the development of dementia and, in fact, may represent early dementia, particularly Alzheimer's disease.

Other associations exist between dementia and depression. Epidemiological studies reveal that depression occurring at any age is associated with an almost two-fold increase in risk of developing dementia, particularly Alzheimer's disease. It is unclear whether depression represents an early symptom arising from common neuropathological processes or an independent risk factor for the development of dementia. The timing of depression onset, in early or late life, may help to determine the link between these two diseases. Depression occurring in the decades before the onset of dementia

suggests depression as a risk factor, as it would be an unlikely early manifestation of dementia so many years in advance. Conversely, depression occurring in the 1–2 years before the onset of dementia suggests depression as an early symptom of dementia, particularly in an individual with no prior history of depression. Evidence exists in support of both hypotheses and there is no agreement at this point. Given what is known about the connection between depression and dementia, it is important to monitor cognition in older patients who have experienced depression at any point in their life.

> ### EVIDENCE AT A GLANCE
>
> Depression occurring at any age is associated with an almost two-fold increase in risk of developing dementia.

The biological basis for these associations remains hypothetical. Proposed pathways linking depression with dementia include vascular disease, hippocampal atrophy, and proinflammatory changes. Because hippocampal atrophy is a hallmark of Alzheimer's disease, researchers have examined hippocampal volume in patients with depression. One study found reduced hippocampal size in patients with recurrent depression with a volume loss that was proportionate to the total duration of depressive symptoms.

One theory of depression is that the hypothalamic-pituitary axis is overactive, which results in chronically elevated levels of cortisol and damage to hippocampal neurons. In support of this theory, a recent study in rats demonstrated hippocampal neuronal damage associated with exogenous administration of corticosterone. Some studies in humans have shown a similar relationship between endogenous cortisol levels, hippocampal volume loss, and memory deficits. Though an appealing hypothesis, studies have been inconsistent in establishing these associations. An alternative hypothesis thus proposes that early amyloid deposition in the hippocampus due to Alzheimer's disease leads to hippocampal atrophy and subsequent depressive symptoms, implicating depression as a prodromal symptom of dementia as opposed to a risk factor. Along these lines, depression may be directly linked to dementia through Alzheimer's disease-specific pathology. Amyloid plaques and neurofibrillary tangles are present in higher amounts in the hippocampus of patients with Alzheimer's disease with a history of major depressive disorder, compared with patients with Alzheimer's disease without a history of depression.

As with depression and Alzheimer's disease, the relationship between depression, vascular disease, and vascular dementia is complex. Vascular pathology has been shown to contribute to cognitive changes as well as dementia, offering support to the connected relationship between depression and dementia. The vascular depression hypothesis, first introduced in 1997 by George Alexopoulos, postulates that cerebrovascular disease is a major contributing factor in late onset depression through disruption of prefrontal systems or their modulating pathways. This can occur with a single lesion or an accumulation of lesions. Support for this hypothesis includes the high prevalence of depression in patients with vascular risk factors, such as diabetes and heart disease; the high prevalence of depression in patients with preexisting cerebrovascular disease, including those who have had symptomatic and asymptomatic strokes; and high prevalence of depression in those with substantial deep white matter lesions. Fujikawa et al. reported that clinically silent cerebral infarcts were found in 93.7% of patients with late onset depression.

In summary, no single process can yet fully explain the neurobiological association between depression and dementia. Depression is a heterogeneous disorder, with contributions from the biological, psychological, and social realms. The processes described are probably not mutually exclusive, and there may be yet undiscovered factors at play. The interaction may be synergistic, with the expression of cognitive impairment dependent on the mix of pathology present in each individual.

Biopsychosocial factors that may contribute to geriatric depression

As noted previously, medical conditions are risk factors for depression, particularly if functional impairment is present. Substance use disorders, such as alcohol dependence, are also associated with depression in old age. Genetic studies have not found any strong markers for late-life depression. No association has been found between the epsilon 4 allele of the apolipoprotein E gene and depressive

symptoms. As with younger populations, female gender, a personal history of depression, and a family history of depression are risk factors for geriatric depression.

From a psychological perspective, individuals with a premorbid personality disorder are four times as likely to experience symptoms of depression as those without. In addition, studies that examine personality traits of older patients with and without depression have suggested that qualities such as hopelessness, rumination (repetitively focusing on a particular thought or set of thoughts), catastrophizing (viewing a situation as considerably worse than it is), less positive reappraisal (focusing on the good in what is happening or has happened), and perception of a lack of self-efficacy (the belief that one is capable of performing successfully in a particular situation) increase risk of depression. Depression may also occur as a result of receiving the diagnosis of Alzheimer's disease or as a reaction to cognitive decline.

A variety of social factors are associated with an increased risk of depression and are prevalent in the aging population. Being unmarried, bereaved, poor, experiencing stressful life events or limited social support, and functional impairment are well-established risk factors for depression in late life.

CASE CONTINUED

Mr S's wife brought him back to the clinic 3 years later, and reported to the primary care provider that Mr S "has been sitting around the house not doing much, I think he is depressed again." He had discontinued sertraline. He interacted less than at previous clinic appointments and deferred most questions to his wife. He denied feeling depressed and acknowledged a preference to just spend his time watching television. His primary care provider again prescribed sertraline, but over 6 months there was little improvement in his function. His wife reported that he was having difficulty with memory, and had made several recent errors in managing the household finances. Cognitive testing was notable for adequate effort but deficits in delayed verbal recall and visual spatial ability. Labwork was unremarkable, with normal serum chemistries, complete blood count, vitamin B12 level, thyroid-stimulating hormone level, and free thyroxine (T4) level. A computed tomography (CT) of the brain was performed as part of the routine work-up and was notable for changes consistent with mild small vessel ischemic disease.

Apathy versus depression

Apathy is derived from the Greek word *pathos*, which means passion. Apathy, therefore, translates to a lack of passion and is described as a loss of motivation associated with diminished function in emotional, cognitive, and behavioral domains. Apathy can be a symptom of depression but is commonly found in dementing disorders in the absence of depression. Because of overlap in appearance and context, distinguishing apathy from depression can confound clinicians. Patients with apathy, however, typically demonstrate a reduced level of initiative, emotional blunting, and a lack of interest in activities. In contrast, loss of interest, psychomotor slowing, and a restricted range of affect are characteristic symptoms of major depression. Apathy in dementia is usually a complaint of the caregiver, not the patient. In fact, patients with apathy rarely seem concerned by their own lack of interest or desire to be active or social. In comparison, patients with depression usually complain of loss of interest or ability to experience pleasure, which is called anhedonia and is distressing to them. Major depressive disorder, in contrast to apathy, is accompanied by a number of other symptoms, including anxiety, depressed mood, changes in sleep and appetite, and feelings of guilt, hopelessness, or shame.

☆ TIPS AND TRICKS

Apathy in dementia is usually a complaint of the caregiver and not the patient. Apathetic patients are frequently not concerned about this lack of initiative and motivation. Patients with major depressive disorder, in contrast, are aware of their lack of interest in previously pleasurable activities. Depression is accompanied by other symptoms including low mood as well as sleep and appetite changes.

Apathy is observed in up to 72% of patients with Alzheimer's disease, but also in a variety of other disease states including schizophrenia, frontotemporal dementia, cerebrovascular disease, human immunodeficiency virus/acquired immune deficiency syndrome, and Parkinson's disease. Apathy in dementia is associated with older age, and more rapid cognitive and functional decline. The differential diagnosis of apathy in dementia should include depression, medication effects (particularly antipsychotics and sedative-hypnotics), stroke (particularly if sudden in onset), hypoactive delirium, and frontal lobe dysfunction. Apathy may be more common in certain types of dementia, particularly the behavioral variant of frontotemporal dementia.

Researchers have developed and validated several scales to quantify apathy among patients with dementia. For example, the Apathy Evaluation Scale consists of 18 questions which assess change in three areas – observable activity, thought content, and emotional reactivity. There are three versions, one for use by the patient, one for use by an informant, and one for use by the clinician.

The evidence base for effective treatment of apathy in dementia is sparse, though there are case reports, open-label trials, and small, randomized placebo-controlled trials that support the use of antidepressants, psychostimulants, and cholinesterase inhibitors. Some experts have recommended that the choice of pharmacological treatment should be guided by the domain most impaired – antidepressants for significant loss of emotional reactivity, psychostimulants for diminished goal-directed behavior, and cholinesterase inhibitors for diminished goal-directed cognition.

Clinical approach to diagnosis of depression in the elderly

Expert debate about the utility of traditional depression criteria as established by the *Diagnostic and Statistical Manual of Mental Disorders*, 4th edition (DSM-IV) and the *International Classification of Diseases*, 10th revision (ICD-10) in geriatric populations has centered around the classification of symptoms that may be attributed to other geriatric illnesses and the difficulty some elderly patients with cognitive impairment have in describing mood when they lack insight into their affective state.

Box 5.2 Atypical presentation of depression in older adults

Denial of depressed mood or sadness
Anxiety and worry, with a focus on physical complaints
Hopelessness
Irritability and/or restlessness
Memory complaints
Lack of interest in personal care
Social withdrawal

☆ TIPS AND TRICKS

The GDS can be useful in assessing for depression in older patients. It is quick to administer, consists of a series of "yes or no" questions, is available in both a long and a short form and can, in general, be self-administered by patients with mild dementia. The GDS becomes less reliable and valid as severity of dementia progresses.

Clinicians may overlook depression in the elderly if it presents atypically with symptoms not covered by the traditional DSM-IV criteria (see Boxes 5.1 and 5.2). Subjectively, depressed older patients may focus on physical symptoms such as dizziness, headache, and fatigue. Anxiety and psychotic symptoms, including delusions of guilt, nihilism (a sense that everything is unreal), or persecution (belief that one is being attacked, harassed, or conspired against) may be so prominent that depressed mood is not noticed. Objectively, the diagnosis may be aided when the clinician observes irritability, social withdrawal, and isolation as indicators of depression.

Screening tools such as the GDS can be helpful. The GDS is available in 15- and 30-item formats, can be self-administered, and consists of "yes or no" questions which inquire about the patient's perspective on their life over the previous week. Physical symptoms that could be related to co-morbid medical conditions are deliberately not assessed. Sensitivity and specificity for major depressive disorder can be as high as 84% and 95%, respectively, when using a score of 11 or more on the 30-item test. Patients with mild dementia are generally able to complete the GDS but it is rendered less valid as levels of cognitive impairment increase. The Cornell Scale for Depression in Dementia, which was developed specifically to assess for depression in patients with dementia, is longer and more time consuming. Information is gathered through two semi-structured interviews, with an informant and with the patient. Sensitivity and specificity for major depressive disorder have been reported to be up to 90% and 75%, respectively.

There are many medical conditions associated with depressive symptomatology, including, but not limited to, cerebrovascular disease, heart disease, cancer, diabetes, and neurological disease such as Parkinson's disease; it is important to screen for depression in these patients. Potentially reversible causes include vitamin B12 deficiency, thyroid disease, medications, and alcohol use. Many of these disorders can also cause or contribute to cognitive impairment. Additionally, hypoactive delirium can present with depressive-like symptoms, and should be considered in any patient who presents with an acute change in behavior or mental status. Other symptoms of delirium include fluctuating levels of consciousness, attention, and cognition, which are not seen in depression.

The evaluation of depression should include a thorough history, as well as a targeted medical and neurological exam. Because of the relationship with dementia, cognitive screening should be included as a standard part of every evaluation of depression. A complete blood cell count, chemistry panel, thyroid function tests, and serum vitamin B12 levels are included as part of a standard evaluation for patients presenting for the first time with depression. Additional labwork should be guided by the history and exam, and might include neuroimaging, liver function tests, urinalysis, and a urine drug screen.

Assessment of suicidal ideation is imperative when depressive symptoms are reported. Twenty percent of all suicide deaths in the United States occur in those older than 65 years, which is substantial given that the elderly account for only about 13% of the population. Men over the age of 69 years have the highest rate of completed suicide. Though moderate-to-severe dementia may protect against suicide, early dementia may pose a risk depending on a person's reaction to the diagnosis and fears about the course of the illness. Data on the rate of suicide in populations with dementia are limited. Studies suggest that typical risk factors (e.g. past psychiatric hospitalizations, history of self-harm) may not always be seen in completed suicides in the elderly and it is not known whether the suicides were related to psychiatric symptoms that were underrecognized or due to some aspect of the dementia itself.

Many suicide researchers report that elderly people have had contact with a healthcare professional, usually a primary care provider, shortly before the act of suicide. Among patients with depression, detecting suicidal ideation can be done directly by asking, "Have you had thoughts of taking your life?" If a patient answers positively to this question, the providers should ask whether or not the patient has developed a plan for self-harm, whether they intend to carry it through, and if they have the means to do so. In general, a patient considered to be at imminent risk (e.g. likely to attempt suicide in the next 2 days) should be hospitalized. If possible, family should be involved and access to potential means of suicide, such as firearms, should be removed. If suicide is not imminent, the patient should be referred to a psychiatrist for evaluation and treatment of psychiatric illness, if present, and an in-depth assessment of contributing psychological and social factors.

⚠ CAUTION

All patients with depression should be assessed for suicidal risk. Consider hospitalizing patients who are at imminent risk for suicidal self-harm. Involve family and limit access to potential means of suicide.

Management of depression in patients with dementia

Treatment of depression can result in an improvement in other dementia-related behavioral symptoms. Antidepressant medications are the mainstay of treatment of depression though the available evidence is mixed for the effectiveness of these medications in treating depression in patients with dementia (Table 5.1). A randomized, placebo-controlled trial published in 2011, comparing mirtazapine, sertraline, and placebo in patients with depression and Alzheimer's disease, did not show any benefit in the treatment arms over placebo in patients followed over 39 weeks, though all patients in the study showed improvement. The American Psychiatric Association practice guideline states, "Although evidence for antidepressant efficacy in patients with dementia and depression is mixed, clinical consensus supports a trial of an antidepressant to treat clinically significant, persistent depressed mood." Low starting doses and small dose increases are recommended. Depression may require more time to remit than in younger patients, and 6–8 weeks should separate dose increases. With dementia progression, the need for ongoing antidepressant treatment may diminish, particularly in patients with Alzheimer's dementia. The treating clinicians should consider stopping antidepressant treatment as the dementia progresses.

EVIDENCE AT A GLANCE

Large, well-done, placebo-controlled randomized trials of antidepressants in patients with both depression and dementia do not support clinical benefit. Clinical consensus, however, supports a trial of an antidepressant to treat clinically significant and persistent depressed mood.

Selective serotonin reuptake inhibitors (SSRI) are generally well tolerated and should be considered first in treating depression in dementia. Several considerations should be taken into account before choosing which SSRI to prescribe. Drug interactions are common with fluoxetine, paroxetine, and fluvoxamine, because of cytochrome P450 enzyme inhibition. Additionally, fluoxetine is generally avoided in the elderly because of its long half-life and paroxetine because of its relatively high affinity for muscarinic acetylcholine receptors compared to other SSRIs. The US Food and Drug Administration recently issued a warning for citalopram, recommending doses no greater than 20 mg in older patients because of the risk of dose-dependent QT interval prolongation. Newer antidepressants, such as venlafaxine, bupropion, and duloxetine, are not well studied in the elderly. Bupropion has been associated with seizures at high doses. Mirtazapine, a tetracyclic

Table 5.1 Pharmacological management of depression

Drug	Starting dose	Maximum dose	Adverse effects	Notes
SSRI				
Sertraline	25 mg	200 mg	GI upset, tremor, hyponatremia, headache	
Citalopram	10 mg	20 mg	GI upset, tremor, QT prolongation, hyponatremia	Recent FDA warning re QT prolongation
Escitalopram	5 mg	10 mg	GI upset, tremor, hyponatremia	
Paroxetine	5 mg	40 mg	GI upset, tremor, hyponatremia	Multiple drug interactions, anticholinergic
Fluoxetine	5 mg	40 mg	GI upset, tremor, hyponatremia	Drug interactions, long half-life
Fluvoxamine	25 mg	300 mg, divided	GI upset, tremor, hyponatremia	Multiple drug interactions, generally avoided
SNRI				
Duloxetine	30 mg	60 mg	GI upset, tremor, hyponatremia, elevated BP	Avoid if hepatic impairment
Venlafaxine	75 mg	375 mg, divided	GI upset, elevated BP, hyponatremia	Available in XR single daily dosing, reduce dose in renal impairment
Other				
Bupropion	75 mg	375 mg	Anxiety, insomnia, seizures, elevated BP	Available in XR single daily dosing, hepatic and renal dosing required
Mirtazapine	7.5 mg	45 mg	Sedation, weight gain, neutropenia	

BP, blood pressure; FDA, Food and Drug Administration; GI, gastrointestinal; SNRI, serotonin-norepinephrine reuptake inhibitor; SSRI, selective serotonin reuptake inhibitor; XR, extended release.

antidepressant that exerts its effect by enhancement of serotonergic neurotransmission, is commonly prescribed for depression in patients with dementia, and treats anxiety, insomnia, and poor appetite. Tricyclic antidepressants are avoided because of cardiac side-effects, orthostasis, and moderate-to-severe anticholinergic properties which are particularly prominent with the tertiary amine tricyclics such as imipramine and amitriptyline.

> **⚕ CAUTION**
>
> Tricyclic antidepressants should be avoided in the elderly because of cardiac side-effects, orthostasis, and anticholinergic properties.

Electroconvulsive therapy (ECT) is the most effective intervention for treating depression, with response rates as high as 90%. It can be helpful for some patients with pseudodementia. Patients are placed under general anesthesia before delivery of a seizure-inducing electrical stimulus. Typically, ECT is delivered 2–3 times a week over the course of several weeks. Anterograde and retrograde memory loss is a common side-effect. Postictal confusion and delirium with ECT may be more significant for patients with dementia. ECT is not well studied in patients with dementia, and use should be reserved for patients with severe symptoms of depression. ECT requires referral to a psychiatrist who is certified in performing the procedure.

SCIENCE REVISITED

ECT is the most effective intervention for treating severe depression in the elderly, and works by inducing seizures in patients while under general anesthesia.

Psychosocial interventions for both patients and family members can be useful in treating depression in patients with dementia. Stimulation-oriented approaches, such as recreational activities including art, music, and dance, and emotion-oriented treatments such as reminiscence therapy and validation therapy, have been shown to improve depression in some studies. Most of these studies were based on small samples, though some were randomized and placebo controlled in design. Frustration, agitation, and depression have been reported as adverse reactions to some types of therapy, particularly those with a cognitive-oriented approach, underscoring the importance of individualizing treatment to the patient's cognitive abilities and frustration tolerance. For example, more structured therapy such as cognitive behavioral therapy and interpersonal therapy are not as effective in patients with cognitive dysfunction because of impairment in language and reasoning.

Finally, family involvement greatly enhances any plan for management of depression in dementia. Yet caregiving can be a burden physically, mentally, and emotionally, with an increase in depression and manifest frustration in the caregiver. Caregiver burnout increases the risk of neglect and out-of-home placement for the care recipient. Monitoring for signs of caregiver burnout and referring family members to sources of care and support can improve the caregiver's depression, overall well-being and ability to care for their loved one.

CASE CONTINUED

Mr S was diagnosed with Alzheimer's dementia and prescribed a cholinesterase inhibitor. He continued to exhibit a gradual decline in cognitive function as well as impairment in independent activities of daily living, ultimately requiring placement in a care facility.

Further reading

Aalten P, de Vugt ME, Jaspers N, et al. The course of neuropsychiatric symptoms in dementia. Part I: findings from the two-year longitudinal Maasbed study. *J Geriatr Psychiatry* 2005; **20**: 523–30.

Banerjee S, Hellier J, Dewey M, et al. Sertraline or mirtazapine for depression in dementia (HTA-SADD): a randomised, multicenter, double-blind, placebo-controlled trial. *Lancet* 2011; **378**: 403–11.

Cereseto M, Reines A, Ferrero A, Sifonios L, Rubio M, Wikinski S. Chronic treatment with high doses of corticosterone decreases cytoskeletal proteins in the rat hippocampus. *Eur J Neurosci* 2006; **24**: 3354–64.

Cho MJ, Lyo IK, Lee DW, et al. Brain single photon emission computed tomography findings in depressive pseudodementia patients. *J Affect Disord* 2002; **69**: 159–66.

Constantine GL, Lourdes D, Steinberg M, et al. Treating depression in Alzheimer disease: efficacy and safety of sertraline therapy, and the benefits of depression reduction: the DIADS. *Arch Gen Psychiatry* 2003; **60**: 737–46.

Drijgers RL, Aalten P, Winogrodzka A. Pharmacological treatment of apathy in neurodegenerative diseases: a systematic review. *Dement Geriatr Cogn Disord* 2009; **28**: 13–22.

Fujikawa T, Yokota N, Muraoka M, Yamawaki S. Incidence of silent cerebral infarction in patients with major depression. *Stroke* 1993; **24**: 1631–4.

Hales RE. *The American Psychiatric Publishing Textbook of Psychiatry*, 5th edn. Arlington, VA: American Psychiatric Publishing, 2008.

Lyketsos CG, Steele C, Baker L, et al. Major and minor depression in Alzheimer's disease:

prevalence and impact. *J Neuropsychiatr Clin Neurosci* 1997; **9**: 556–61.

Madden JJ, Luhan JA, Kaplan LA, Manfredi HM. Nondementing psychoses in older persons. *JAMA* 1952; **16**: 1567–70.

Mega MS, Cummings JL, Fiorello T, et al. The spectrum of behavioral changes in Alzheimer's disease. *Neurology* 1996; **46**: 130–5.

National Institute of Mental Health. *Older Adults: Depression and Suicide Facts*. NIH Publication No. 4593. Bethesda, MD: National Institutes of Health, 2007.

Payne JL, Sheppard JM, Steinberg M, et al. Incidence, prevalence, and outcomes of depression in residents of a long-term care facility with dementia. *Int J Geriatr Psychiatry* 2002; **17**: 247–53.

Pearlson GD, Rabins PV, Kim WS, et al. Structural brain CT changes and cognitive deficits in elderly depressives with and without reversible dementia (pseudodementia). *Psychol Med* 1989; **19**: 573–84.

Sheline YI, Wang PW, Gado MH, Csernansky JG, Vannier MW. Hippocampal atrophy in recurrent major depression. *Proc Natl Acad Sci USA* 1996; **30**: 3908–13.

6

Mild Cognitive Impairment

Ranjan Duara,[1,2,3] **David A. Loewenstein,**[1,2] **Clinton Wright,**[2] **Elizabeth Crocco**[2] **and Daniel Varon**[1,3]

[1]Wien Center for Alzheimer's Disease and Memory Disorders, Mount Sinai Medical Center, USA
[2]Departments of Neurology and Psychiatry and Behavioral Sciences, University of Miami, Miller School of Medicine, USA
[3]Department of Neurology, Herbert Wertheim College of Medicine, Florida International University, USA

Introduction

Most diseases go through a transitional stage (e.g. "pre-diabetes" and "pre-hypertension") before they develop the clinical features that are required to fulfill established criteria for the diagnosis to be made with reasonable certainty. It is becoming increasingly important to introduce treatment for slowly progressive diseases at an earlier stage, so that treatment may have a greater impact and prevent or slow transition to more severe stages of the disease. Currently, disease-modifying treatments are not available for degenerative diseases of the brain, which are the main etiological factor for mild cognitive impairment (MCI) and dementia. Effective treatments are presently available to prevent cerebrovascular damage and interventions for such modifiable risk factors may modify the course of the disease, by preventing new vascular lesions from developing. Thus, secondary prevention remains the major option for providing a measurable therapeutic impact on the underlying disease, by earlier detection at the MCI (or even earlier) stage. The goals of this chapter, therefore, are to enable clinicians to: (a) recognize and diagnose MCI and its cognitive subtypes, (b) diagnose the likely etiology of MCI syndromes, (c) understand the risk factors for and modes of progression, and (d) be informed about optimal methods available for treatment and prevention of progression of MCI syndromes.

Definition

The term mild cognitive impairment was first described by Reisberg in 1982 as a condition associated with an increased risk of progression to dementia. It was, however, the Mayo Criteria for MCI published by Petersen et al[1,2]. which resulted in widespread use of this term. Originally designed for the diagnosis of a pre-Alzheimer disease condition, the term MCI is now widely used to describe the predementia phase of any disease that may ultimately progress to a dementia syndrome.

> **PETERSEN'S CRITERIA FOR MILD COGNITIVE IMPAIRMENT**
>
> 1. Memory complaints, preferably corroborated by an informant.
> 2. Evidence of objective memory impairment for the age of the patient, as assessed by neuropsychological testing (most frequently assessed using tests such as the Memory for Passages-Delayed Recall from the Wechsler Memory Scale, the list

Dementia, First Edition. Edited by Joseph F. Quinn.
© 2014 John Wiley & Sons, Ltd. Published 2014 by John Wiley & Sons, Ltd.

learning test of the ADAS-Cog or the Rey Auditory Verbal Learning Test.

3. Preserved global cognition (most frequently established by a Mini-Mental State Exam (MMSE) score of 26/30 or greater.
4. Essentially intact activities of daily living (ADLs).
5. Absence of dementia.

Grundman et al[3]. have proposed an adaptation of Petersen's criteria, to improve reliability when these criteria are used in clinical trials, as follows:

1) memory complaints to be corroborated by an informant
2) abnormal memory functioning on the Logical Memory II subtest of the Wechsler Memory Scale
3) normal general cognitive functioning based on clinical judgment and an MMSE score of 24/30 or greater 4. no or minimal impairment in function (i.e. a Clinical Dementia Rating global score of 0.5).

These adapted criteria may be operationalized for general clinical use, as shown in Table 6.1.

Mild cognitive impairment subtypes

The heterogeneity of MCI is a consequence of a number of factors, which include the methodology used to classify MCI, the underlying etiology of the MCI syndrome and the premorbid state of the patient, including the level of education, cultural background and the general medical, neurological, and psychiatric status. Broadly, MCI may be classified according to the predominant form of cognitive impairment (i.e. amnestic or non-amnestic MCI), the suspected etiology (e.g. Alzheimer's disease, vascular cognitive impairment, Lewy body disease) or the progression rates of cognitive deficits (e.g. progressive versus non-progressive, or even reversible MCI). Amnestic and non-amnestic MCI may each be further subdivided into single or multiple domain MCI. Multidomain amnestic MCI (aMCI) requires impairment in memory and one or more non-memory domains; multidomain non-amnestic MCI (naMCI) requires impairment in two or more non-memory domains, such as attention/executive functioning, language, and visuospatial processing.

Table 6.1 Criteria for amnestic mild cognitive impairment

Formal criteria	Operationalization of formal criteria in clinical practice
Memory complaint, preferably corroborated by an informant	Interview with informant
Objective memory impairment for age and education	Score below age and education cut-off on neuropsychological test (e.g. logical memory II subscale [delayed paragraph recall] from the Wechsler Memory Scale)
Largely intact general cognitive function	Mini-Mental State Examination score between 24 and 30 (inclusive)
Essentially preserved activities of daily living	Cognition and functional capacity not sufficiently impaired for a diagnosis of dementia
Not demented	Clinical Dementia Rating of 0.5

Reproduced from Petersen et al[4]. with permission from Lippincott Williams and Wilkins.

Impairments in episodic memory occur not uncommonly in conjunction with other cognitive deficits. A purely amnestic form of MCI occurs in approximately one-third of MCI cases, and the largest single MCI group is characterized by impairment in memory and one or more non-memory domains.

Longitudinal studies in memory disorder clinics have demonstrated a rate of progression from MCI to Alzheimer's disease (AD) of 12–15% per year, with a low rate of reversal (less than 5% per year) while community-based epidemiological studies demonstrate a lower rate of conversion (5–10% per year) and higher rates of reversal (up to 25% per year). These findings suggest that factors other than cognitive test performance *per se*, such as subtle impairment of functional ability observed by family members and friends or colleagues at work, are a strong determinant of the future rate of progression.

Conditions such as AD, Lewy body disease (LBD), frontotemporal lobar dementia (FTLD), and vascular dementia (VaD) may present with MCI and gradually transition to a dementia state. It is important to recognize that in these diseases MCI represents a wide spectrum of cognitive and very subtle functional impairments, rather than a point in the progression from normal aging to dementia. Reversible causes of MCI, such as anxiety states, attentional disorders, depression, metabolic and nutritional disorders and medication side-effects, are usually subacute in onset and may often be superimposed on, and may unmask the features of, underlying degenerative or vascular pathology. Accordingly, it is not unusual for an initial cognitive and functional response to management of these reversible conditions to be followed by gradual cognitive and functional decline.

Pathophysiology

A transitional, predementia state, between normal cognition and established dementia, is likely to exist for most recognizable dementing disorders The use of different criteria for diagnosing MCI may result in MCI prevalence rates of 1–3% of the population over 65 years of age. Nevertheless, regardless of the criteria used, patients diagnosed with MCI have been found to have a high likelihood of progression to dementia and often to Alzheimer's disease.

The most well-studied pathological entity that results in an MCI syndrome is AD. Pathological changes associated with this disease may be present a decade or more before the onset of clinical symptoms and signs, and include the deposition of amyloid beta protein in the neocortex. Although amyloid deposition itself may result in subtle cognitive deficits, it is the neurodegenerative phase of AD which results in the deficits in delayed memory characteristic of this disease. Deficits on delayed recall tests are caused by neurodegenerative involvement of the medial temporal structures such as the entorhinal cortex (ERC) and the CA1 sector and subiculum of the hippocampus (HP).

Three clinical phases have been suggested to describe the progression of AD: (a) a presymptomatic stage in which initial pathological changes occur without clinical manifestations; (b) a prodromal stage characterized by cognitive deficits not severe enough to warrant a diagnosis of dementia (MCI); and (c) a symptomatic stage in which dementia can be clearly diagnosed. During the presymptomatic stage, amyloid deposition appears to initiate the development of neurofibrillary tangles in the transentorhinal and entorhinal cortex (ERC), the hippocampus (HP), limbic system and eventually the neocortex, leading in time to synaptic dysfunction, cell death, and brain atrophy.

The plasticity of the brain and the effects of cognitive reserve (see below) allow some patients with advanced pathological stages of the disease (i.e. Braak stage V or VI) to escape cognitive symptoms and functional deficits. In fact, in one study about 30% of individuals who met neuropathological criteria for AD at autopsy were considered non-demented during life. In another longitudinal study, almost all patients classified as MCI during life were found to have neurodegenerative pathology at autopsy. In about 30% of these cases, pathologies other than AD, such as Lewy bodies, argyrophilic grain disease, hippocampal sclerosis and/or cerebrovascular disease, are present.

The concept of vascular cognitive impairment (VCI) has evolved over several decades as advancements in brain computed tomography (CT) and especially magnetic resonance imaging (MRI) have allowed greater detection of vascular damage. Because vascular disease is prevalent in older people , vascular lesions are often co-mingled with Alzheimer pathology. The concept of VaMCI has also evolved because subclinical vascular damage, such as white matter lesions, infarcts, and microhemorrhages, have been found to associate with cognitive consequences, even in the absence of a clinical event, such as a stroke. Evidence from large population-based studies has shown that subclinical vascular damage is associated with a spectrum of cognitive deficits ranging from subtle changes to

MCI (manifesting often as executive dysfunction, rather than an amnestic disorder) to dementia.

Vascular insults are an important cause of and contributor to the development of VaMCI, although the volume and location of tissue both necessary and sufficient to cause such impairment have not been established. For example, small "strategic" infarcts in the anterior thalamus and other areas can produce amnestic disorders of varying severity, and small infarcts in other locations can produce deficits corresponding to the functions attributable to those regions. However, both the volume and the number of infarcts are known to be associated with the risk of dementia. Likewise, the volume of white matter lesions necessary to cause VaMCI or VaD is unknown. However, community-based data show that both Alzheimer and vascular pathology are prevalent and that each contributes to cognitive performance in those with MCI that reach autopsy.

The presence, severity, and type of cognitive impairment in a given individual depend not only on the location, severity, and type of pathology present in the brain, but also on the resilience of that individual to withstand the effects of that pathology. This resilience is known, broadly, as cognitive reserve and is associated with various factors that can be subdivided as "pure" cognitive reserve and "brain reserve." Among those factors related to pure cognitive reserve are the individual's level of education, overall intelligence, occupational attainment, and exposure to information as well as exposure to various stimuli and activities. Factors associated with brain reserve include brain size, age, developmental and premorbid conditions, such as dyslexia and attention deficit disorder, brain trauma, cerebrovascular disease, and systemic illnesses. It is importance to consider cognitive reserve as a major factor determining when and with what severity an individual with a specified brain pathology, such as Alzheimer's disease, will manifest with cognitive symptoms and objective evidence of impairment.

Symptoms mimicking early dementia and impaired performance on cognitive tests may be related to a variety of medical conditions, effects of medications, psychosocial factors, and psychiatric conditions, such as anxiety, depression, and personality disorders. Furthermore, in the early phase of MCI, it may be difficult to distinguish (a) functional impairment associated with normal aging from abnormal aging, especially in the presence of age-related conditions such as arthritis, visual and hearing impairment, and (b) cognitive deficits from the normal age-related cognitive decline, especially among those with high or low cognitive reserve, psychiatric co-morbidity and those with visual or hearing impairments.

★ TIPS AND TRICKS

Symptoms mimicking early dementia and impaired performance on cognitive tests may be related to a variety of medical conditions, effects of medications, psychosocial factors, and psychiatric conditions, such as anxiety, depression, and personality disorders. Always consider these possibilities when you evaluate a patient presenting with mild cognitive impairment.

Neuropsychological assessment

Neuropsychological evaluation is considered an important tool for confirming the diagnosis of MCI and when it is easily available and affordable, neuropsychological assessment is the preferred method of diagnosis. Many clinicians who conduct dementia and cognitive evaluations use combinations of convenient and brief cognitive tests to make an MCI diagnosis. While simple cognitive screening tests, such as the Folstein Mini-Mental State Examination, are useful for distinguishing dementia from a normal cognitive state, they remain insensitive for detecting MCI. Cognitive screening tests that may better distinguish MCI from normal cognition include the Montreal Cognitive Assessment (MoCA) and the Multiple Delayed Recall Test.

★ TIPS AND TRICKS

The Montreal Cognitive Assessment (MoCA) can be an effective tool to briefly screen for MCI in an office setting, showing greater sensitivity than the Folstein MMSE in detecting subtle cognitive impairments.
www.mocatest.org

Neuropsychological tests commonly used to determine performance in domains required to assess MCI include verbal fluency measures, such as the Controlled Oral Word Association Test (COWAT).

Various cut-off scores have been used for these tests, although 1.5 SD below age- and education-adjusted norms, for a single measure, appears to be most effective in identifying MCI. It is also important to consider the ethnic and cultural background of subjects in determining appropriate cut-off scores. The use of multiple measures to identify memory impairment has been suggested to improve reliability. A cut-off score of at least 1.0 SD below mean normative values on at least two cognitive tests in the same cognitive domain is recommended to decrease the false-positive rate in classification.

There appears to be considerable overlap between amnestic and non-amnestic MCI, depending on the criteria and cut-off scores used to classify impairment. The prevalence rates for MCI subtypes will depend on the use of different cut-off scores, the choice of individual tests used to identify impairment and the control group used to derive such cut-off scores. Reducing the threshold for classifying impairment in a memory test from 1.5 to 1.0 SD will have the effect of increasing the frequency of aMCI relative to naMCI. Individuals with high premorbid educational attainment, or cognitive reserve, may be able to compensate for their deficits because of their greater knowledge base and familiarity with the test-taking process and by employing various strategies that allow them to perform well on cognitive measures, in spite of their deficits. Those with low educational levels may perform far worse than expected, not only because of a lower knowledge base but also because of lack of familiarity with test taking and the associated anxiety and attentional problems.

The cognitive assessment of MCI requires the assessment of memory, language, visuospatial skills, and executive function. Suggested measures for each of these domains are presented in Box 6.1.

Biomarkers in mild cognitive impairment

Biomarkers are surrogates of underlying pathology and unlike clinical and neuropsychological assessments, are not subject to influence by various demographic, psychosocial, medical, and psychiatric factors, nor by hearing and visual deficits. An individual may be biomarker positive without necessarily manifesting any cognitive symptoms or deficits. Biomarkers can be useful in diagnosis by identifying the presence of underlying pathology, even in the preclinical stage of diseases such as AD and FTLD. The accumulation of amyloid (Abeta1-42) in the brain suggests the first phase of AD pathology, whereas regional brain atrophy suggests the presence of neurodegenerative pathology in the brain. Besides being useful diagnostically, biomarkers may also predict the rate of progression of the clinical syndrome, because the severity of the underlying pathology, as measured by the biomarker, is often correlated to the rate of clinical progression.

Box 6.1 Recommended neuropsychological measures for assessing MCI				
Hopkins Verbal Learning Test	Boston Naming Test	Wisconsin Card Sorting Test	Block Design (WAIS- R)	Trail Making Test (Part A)
Fuld Object Memory Test	Letter Fluency Test (FAS)	Trail Making Test (Part B)	Visual Reproduction (Copy Condition)	Digit Symbol Subtest (WAIS-IV)
Rey Auditory Learning Test	Category Fluency Test	Similarities Subtest (WAIS-IV)	Hooper Visual Organization Test	
Memory for Passages (Wechsler Memory Scale)				
Visual Reproduction (Wechlser Memory Scale)				

Cerebrospinal fluid (CSF)

Currently the most promising CSF biomarkers for the diagnosis of early AD are the ratio of CSF Abeta levels to tau protein and CSF phosphotau -231 (ptau-231). CSF Abeta1-42 (the 42 amino acid form of Abeta) is an early marker (including the preclinical and MCI stages) of the amyloid phase of the disease. Somewhat paradoxically, CSF Abeta1-42 is lower in individuals with Abeta pathology, starting in the preclinical phase. CSF total tau, i.e. T-tau, is associated with tangle formation and phosphotau is a marker of the later neurodegenerative phase of the disease. Both tau and phosphotau are elevated in CSF of individuals with AD brain pathology. The CSF Abeta-42:tau ratio differentiated patients with subjective cognitive complaints, with naMCI, and with aMCI from healthy controls. CSF biomarkers have also been shown to have utility in predicting cognitive decline in cognitively normal older adults and progression to a MCI state, as well as progression of aMCI to AD. The measurements are commercially available but their use for predictive purposes in asymptomatic or even MCI patients is currently confined to the research setting.

Neuroimaging

Alterations in the structure of the brain can be detected and quantified by several structural imaging techniques, such as computed tomography (CT) and magnetic resonance imaging (MRI), especially in the medial temporal lobes where AD- and FTLD-related degenerative pathology appear to be most prominent early in the disease process. Functional changes in the brain can be assessed with positron emission tomography (PET) and single photon emission computed tomography (SPECT), as well as by functional MRI (fMRI). Amyloid deposition in the brain can be detected using investigational PET scans with either C-11 or F-18 labeled ligands that bind to fibrillar amyloid beta protein. Although FDA approval of amyloid PET imaging appears to be imminent, practice guidelines are not yet established for using these scans for diagnosis or prognosis in MCI patients. Genetic markers, such as APOE genotypes, can identify subgroups of individuals who are at elevated risk for cognitive decline and the development of AD pathology but the value of APOE genotyping for prognosis in individual subjects with MCI (i.e. in clinical practice) remains to be established.

Magnetic resonance imaging

The presence of an underlying pathology that may be related to an MCI syndrome is currently best identified using MRI, because of its high spatial resolution and ability to distinguish tissue types based on biochemical constituency. The absence of pathology and its presence are important in making an accurate clinical diagnosis, although in many age-related diseases, such as vascular or degenerative dementia, non-specific pathological processes may be discovered, which may obfuscate the diagnosis. The most frequent clinical questions that can be answered by MRI include whether or not the findings on the brain images exclude certain diagnoses, such as vascular dementia, normal pressure hydrocephalus (NPH), space-occupying lesions, such as chronic subdural hematoma or a brain tumor, miscellaneous lesions such as amyloid angiopathy and diseases of the white matter. However, the diagnosis of AD, in its MCI or dementia phase, is the most frequent diagnostic entity that clinicians must address, because the prior probability that patients have this condition is relatively high and the most common query from patients or their relatives is whether or not there is any evidence of AD.

Assessment of hippocampal and entorhinal cortex atrophy in structural brain images could be an inclusive test for the diagnosis of prodromal and probable AD. The pathological process in AD begins in medial temporal structures and the density of this pathology has a proportional effect on the degree of atrophy in these structures. Both hippocampal and entorhinal cortex atrophy, as measured by MR imaging, are markers for AD-related pathology among MCI patients. Atrophy of these structures can be measured semi-quantitatively by the clinician using a visual rating scale (Figure 6.1). The severity of atrophy is correlated with the risk for cognitive impairment and for the rate of progression[5], although the onset and progression of the cognitive deficits are also dependent on cognitive and brain reserve capacity, including the presence of vascular brain disease. In the presence of an MCI syndrome of apparently degenerative etiology, the absence of hippocampal and especially entorhinal cortex atrophy suggests an alternative to AD, such as Lewy body dementia, as the etiology.

Rating	Structural changes	MRI
Rating = 0 (No atrophy) Hippocampus (HPC) with no atrophy Entorhinal Cortex (ERC) with no atrophy Collateral Sulcus (CS) shows no widening	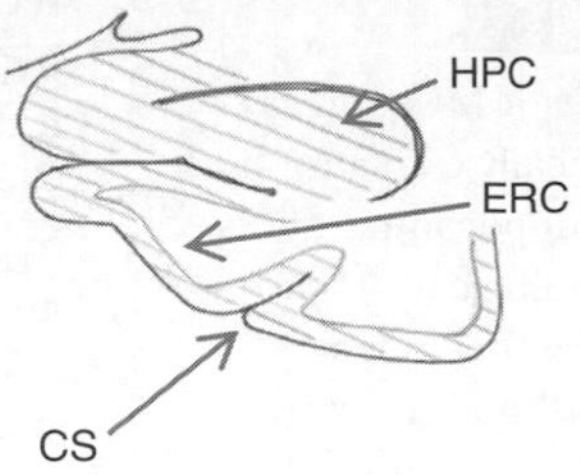	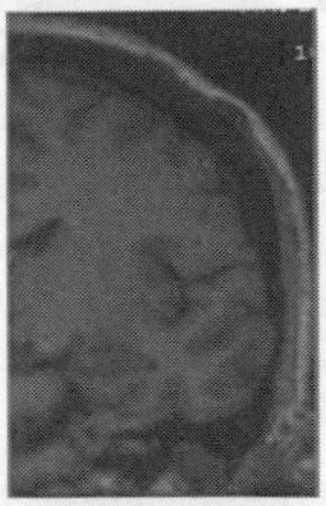
Rating = 1 (Minimal) HPC with less than 25% decrease in thickness. ERC with minimal decreased in thickness or minimal CS widening or both	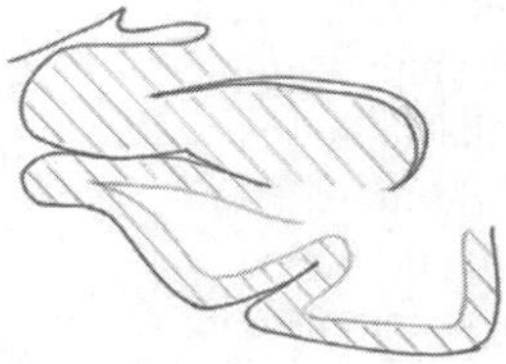	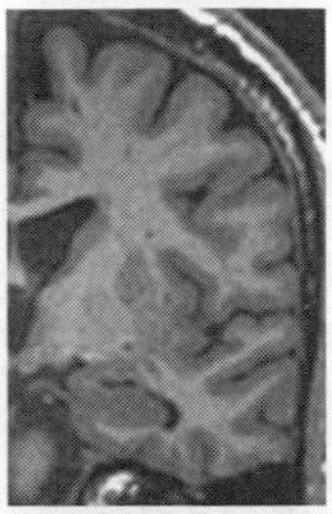
Rating = 2 (Mild) HPC with 25 to 50% decrease in thickness ERC with mild decrease in thickness or mild CS widening or both	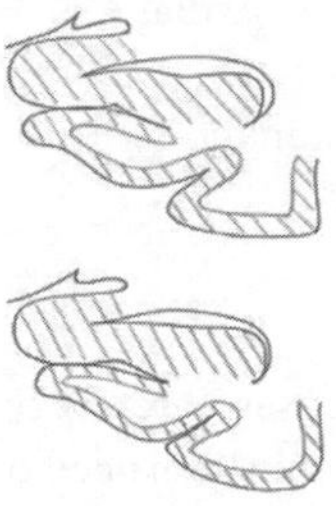	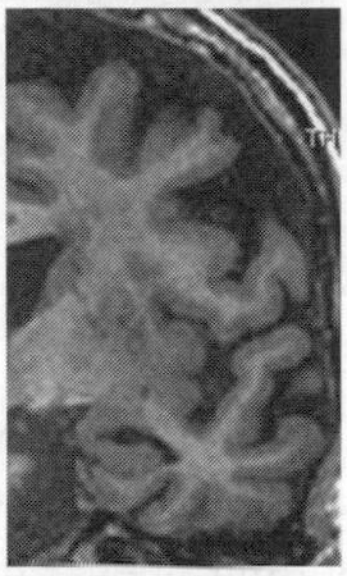
Rating = 3 (Moderate) HPC with 50 to 75% decrease in thickness ERC with moderate decrease in thickness or moderate CS widening or both	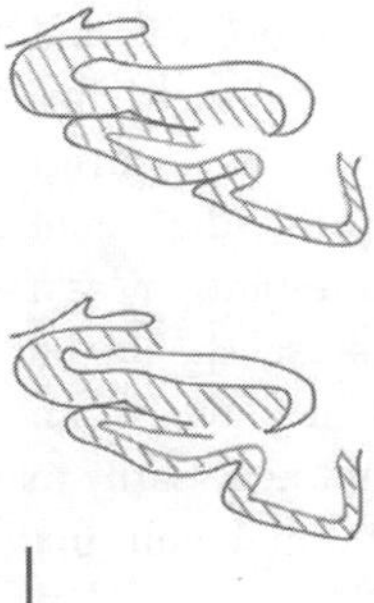	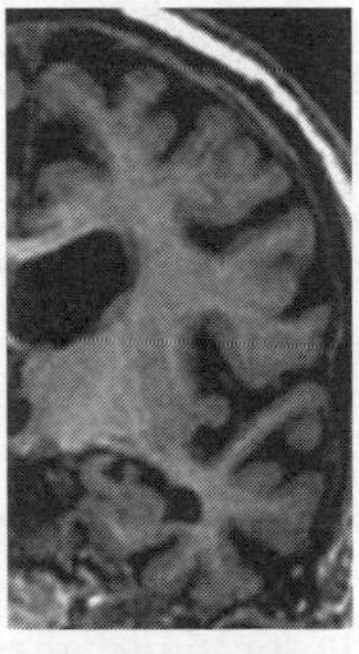
Rating = 4 (Severe) HPC with more than 75% decrease in thickness ERC with severe decrease in thickness and severe widening of collateral sulcus	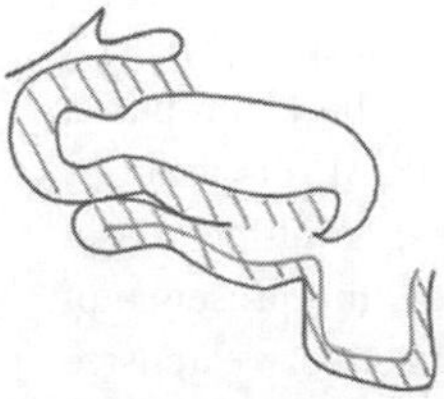	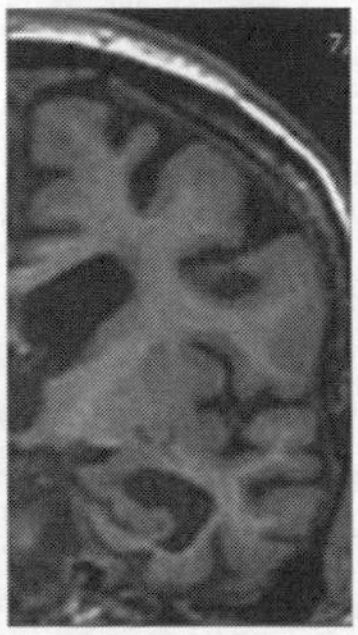

Figure 6.1 Visual rating scale. CS, collateral sulcus; ERC, entorhinal cortex; HPC, hippocampus. Reproduced from Urs et al[2]. with permission from Lippincott Williams and Wilkins.

The presence of both amnestic MCI and AD has been associated specifically with atrophy of the hippocampus, parahippocampal gyrus, and amygdala. Clinicopathological correlations have repeatedly shown that atrophy of these medial temporal structures is correlated with the severity of neurofibrillary tangles, neuritic plaques and the loss of neurons and dendritic arbor in the transentorhinal cortex, and the hippocampus. Although the presence of medial temporal atrophy is not specific for AD (frontotemporal lobar dementia, vascular dementia, and hippocampal sclerosis may also demonstrate brain atrophy in these regions), because of the high prevalence of AD in the elderly, 85–90% of all degenerative pathology in the medial temporal lobe in elderly subjects is AD pathology, either alone or in combination with other diseases.

Vascular and degenerative diseases are very common among the elderly, so it should be expected that MRI evidence of both pathologies will co-exist in many patients. However, in any given case the individual contributions of degenerative and vascular disease to the cognitive impairment may not be easily discernible. Except for cardiac arrest and hypoxic-ischemic encephalopathy, the extent of hippocampal and entorhinal cortex atrophy as a result of pure vascular brain disease should be minimal. Cognitive impairment resulting from vascular brain disease is related not necessarily to the volume of the brain involved by infarctions but to the location of these infarctions.

Magnetic resonance imaging criteria implicating cerebrovascular disease in the etiology of cognitive impairment include a single strategically placed infarction (angular gyrus, thalamus, basal forebrain, or posterior cerebral artery [PCA] or anterior cerebral artery [ACA] territories), multiple basal ganglia and white matter lacunae, the presence of multiple large vessel infarctions, or extensive periventricular white matter lesions, or combinations thereof. Subcortical infarcts appear as cavities that are hypointense on T1 and hyperintense on T2 sequences, and on fluid-attenuated inversion recovery (FLAIR) sequences appear to have a hypointense center and a hyperintense rim around it. However, because many clinical MRIs use 5 mm slices with a 5 mm gap between each slice, discrete hyperintensities seen on FLAIR could be the edge of an infarct rather than a white matter lesion. In addition, microinfarcts are not detected even on 3 Tesla MR scanners but clinicopathological studies suggest that microinfarcts are independent contributors to cognitive disorders even taking into account macroinfarcts. Finally, cerebral microbleeds seen on T2* gradient echo MR sequences suggest either small vessel disease due to chronic hypertension or, if restricted to cerebral cortex, amyloid angiopathy.

Normal pressure hydrocephalus, which is a potentially reversible condition, is important to identify by MRI. However, among elderly individuals, NPH does not usually occur in isolation but in conjunction with degenerative or vascular disease of the brain. Many patients diagnosed on the basis of clinical (cognitive impairment/urinary incontinence and gait disorder) and imaging criteria show an initial benefit after shunting, especially improvement in gait, only to continue to decline cognitively and ultimately with respect to incontinence and gait disorder. Visual rating of MRI scans, assessing enlargement of the perihippocampal fissures (a convenient substitute for assessing medial temporal/hippocampal atrophy), has been shown to be useful in predicting shunt responsiveness.

MRI can be very helpful in identifying the subgroup of patients who do not have significant vascular and, especially, degenerative pathology contributing to the etiology of the NPH syndrome, and in assisting in determining the priority of performing a shunting procedure in a given patient.

Frontotemporal lobar dementia and Alzheimer etiologies for an MCI syndrome have many overlapping features on MRI. Perhaps more than for any other neurodegenerative condition, findings on MRI scan should also take into consideration the age of the subject and clinical syndrome for predicting the underlying etiology. The presence of frontal and anterior, medial, and lateral temporal atrophy, especially if asymmetrical, is suggestive of FTLD, though this is often not sufficiently diagnostic, especially in patients presenting with MCI.

FDG-PET and SPECT scans

Positron emission tomography and SPECT are sensitive methods for providing quantitative evaluation of physiological functions. Radiolabeled glucose FDG (fluoro-2-deoxy-D-glucose)-PET can be used to measure cerebral glucose metabolism, which indirectly indicates synaptic activity. Metabolic or perfusion deficits detected on PET or SPECT scans in AD patients (symmetrical or asymmetrical metabolic deficits in bilateral parietal and temporal lobes) distinguish them from normal control subjects and from patients with other types of dementia. Using FDG-PET, with an automated method of image analysis to study the medial temporal regions and hippocampus, de Leon and colleagues showed that baseline FDG-PET measures predicted decline from normal to MCI or AD, 6–7 years in advance of symptoms with 71% and 81% accuracy, respectively. An extrapolation of these results suggests that AD can be identified 12 years before the patient is symptomatic.

Positron emission tomography scans using FDG measure regional glucose metabolism, which is primarily a biomarker for synaptic activity, while SPECT scans are generally used to measure regional cerebral blood flow. FDG-PET and SPECT scans seem to be the most useful methods to establish a diagnosis of FTLD, when the onset, clinical presentation, or course of cognitive impairment is atypical for AD and FTLD is suspected as an alternative neurodegenerative cause of cognitive decline. Specifically, symptoms such as social disinhibition, awkwardness, difficulties with language, or loss of executive function are more prominent early in the course of FTLD than the memory loss typical of AD. PET and SPECT scans can also be useful for the diagnosis of very early AD when the MRI scan is insufficiently diagnostic or to assist in the diagnosis of other entities such as progressive supranuclear palsy, in which the PET/SPECT scan usually shows a clear demarcation between hypometabolic frontal lobes and normal metabolism in the parietal, temporal, and occipital lobes.

Amyloid PET

Amyloid deposition in the neocortex of the brain may be the earliest detectable biomarker abnormality in early Alzheimer's disease. It has been hypothesized that in the evolution of AD pathology, amyloid deposition is the earliest event, leading to downstream events, including neurodegeneration and cognitive impairment. In the ADNI study it was found that amyloid load increases very early, but tends to plateau much earlier than the rate of loss of brain volume, in what was presumed to be the preclinical and very early clinical stages of AD. The prevalence of positive amyloid scans, using ^{11}C-PIB as the PET ligand, in cognitively apparently healthy volunteers increased rapidly with age, from 6% in 50–59 year olds up to 50% in subjects >80 years of age. Elevated amyloid load in non-demented elderly subjects has been associated with subtle impairment in memory performance, and greater risk for progression to MCI and dementia.

Amyloid PET has not been approved for clinical application by regulatory agencies, as of this writing. If and when it is, the likely clinical application will be primarily to determine evidence of amyloid deposition and risk for cognitive decline among symptomatic individuals with very mild or no objective cognitive impairment or among those with strong risk for dementing diseases, such as a family history of multiple individuals with dementia. Amyloid PET may also be useful for distinguishing FTLD (amyloid negative) from AD (amyloid positive) in the MCI or dementia stage. Currently, a negative amyloid PET scan appears to have more clinical utility than a positive scan. In this regard, among questions that will need to be addressed are: (1) what is the (age-adjusted) threshold for a truly negative and a truly positive amyloid PET scan? and (2) how well do MRI scans that are either positive or negative for neurodegenerative disease compare with PET scans that are amyloid positive or negative?

SCIENCE REVISITED

Biomarkers may be surrogate markers for underlying pathology in the brain such as amyloid deposition or neurodegeneration. Reduced beta amyloid levels in the CSF and elevated cortical amyloid levels on PET are related to the level of amyloid deposition in the brain, while elevated CSF tau levels and atrophic changes in the medial temporal lobes and neocortex on structural MRI are related to neurodegeneration. Hypometabolism of FDG-PET scans is indicative of synaptic loss and/or dysfunction.

Genetic markers

Among the less than 1% of familial dementia cases with an apparent autosomal dominant transmission, a screen for mutations in the presenilin 1 gene (chromosome 14; onset 25–60 years), amyloid precursor protein gene (chromosome 21; onset age 40–70 years) or presenilin 2 gene (chromosome 1; onset 45–84 years) may establish the diagnosis. The most common genetic risk factor for late onset AD, the APOE 4 allele, is associated with a greater prevalence and an earlier age of onset of AD in most racial/ethnic groups. The epsilon 4 allele for the apolipoprotein E (APOE) gene on chromosome 19 is a risk factor that explains about 20% of late onset cases. Those heterozygous for the e4 allele have a 2–3-fold increased risk for AD whereas homozygosity for the e4 allele confers a 10–15-fold increased risk for AD. The presence of the APOE 4 genotype combined with clinical features has been used to increase the predictive accuracy of the diagnosis of AD, especially in its predementia phase.

> **EVIDENCE AT A GLANCE**
>
> Amyloid deposition in the brain occurs to a much greater extent among individuals who are APOE 4 carriers and, especially, those homozygous for the APOE 4 allele. It is presumed that this is the primary mechanism by which risk for AD is increased among individuals who are APOE 4 positive.

Diagnosis of etiological subtypes of mild cognitive impairment

Once a global cognitive diagnosis of MCI or dementia is determined, an etiological diagnosis that is based on the same clinical, neuroimaging, and laboratory features required to make a series of dementia diagnoses may be assigned. Examples of such MCI etiological diagnoses are: MCI-AD (early Alzheimer's disease), VaMCI, MCI-LBD (early Lewy body dementia), MCI-FTD (early frontotemporal dementia), etc. Many of these conditions may result in cognitive impairment without the impairment in social and occupational function that is required for a dementia syndrome and are classified as MCI. Cognitively impaired subjects seen in a memory disorder center are much more likely to have AD than those recruited from a community study. Subjects found to have cognitive impairment in a stroke clinic, renal clinic, cancer center or sleep center are unlikely to be referred for cognitive assessment, because the assumption made, which may often be correct, is that the cognitive impairment is associated either with the major medical condition that the patient is suffering from or its treatment. The availability of neuropsychological evaluation, brain imaging, and CSF evaluation may be determined by prevailing healthcare regulations and regional biases towards the use of certain tests. Figure 6.1 provides a guide to the diagnosis of etiological subtypes of MCI using clinical features and biomarkers.

> **EVIDENCE AT A GLANCE**
>
> In the largest study of its kind to date, autopsy in MCI patients who progressed to dementia revealed that 70% had AD, 9% had LBD, 9% had FTLD and other tauopathies, and only 3% had predominantly vascular pathology. Vascular disease frequently co-existed with other pathologies, including AD.

The accuracy of diagnosis of each MCI subtype remains to be established by longitudinal studies followed to autopsy. Diagnostic accuracy may also be influenced by the specific tests that are used and how they are interpreted (for example, currently it is only the exceptional radiologist who will assess and comment on the severity of medial temporal atrophy on an MRI scan). Diagnostic criteria for the individual causes of dementia generally require the exclusion of all other identifiable neurological, psychiatric, and medical causes of dementia or cognitive impairment. Alzheimer's disease commonly presents as amnestic MCI, whereas conditions such as FTLD or dementia with Lewy bodies are more likely than AD to present initially as naMCI. Nevertheless, no specific cognitive presentation, other than the amnestic subtype, is associated with a specific cause. Etiological subtypes of MCI also can be recognized using established criteria for different forms of dementias, such as AD, LBD, FTLD, and vascular cognitive impairment among non-demented patients.

Patients seen in the hospital or being treated in a specialty clinic are most likely to have MCI as a neurological manifestation of a systemic illness. As such, the dominant medical illnesses present in each individual should be emphasized as possible etiological factors for an MCI syndrome.

MCI-AD

A substantial subgroup of MCI patients who progress to dementia develop AD. While these patients usually present with memory deficits, other presentations are not infrequent, including those who develop deficits in language (primary progressive aphasia), executive or visual-spatial function and those who present with frontal lobe syndromes, such as apathy or disinhibition. Nevertheless, it has been shown that a targeted clinical history alone, providing evidence of cognitive and functional decline relative to previously attained abilities, can identify non-demented subjects who will progress and be found to have histopathological AD on autopsy. The items in the history that best predict future development of AD can be summarized in a simple questionnaire, known as the AD8. The best cognitive biomarker of AD, in its predementia state, appears to be impairment of episodic memory even among asymptomatic, community-dwelling elders.

MRI, parietotemporal deficits of PET or SPECT scanning or abnormal CSF analysis of amyloid beta or tau proteins)[7]. Classification of "preclinical AD" and MCI due to AD has been proposed by work groups convened by the National Institute on Aging and the Alzheimer's Association (NIA-AA criteria) (www.alz. org/research/diagnostic criteria). They issued their recommendations for new diagnostic criteria for Alzheimer's disease based on the following proposed clinicopathological stages of predementia AD. The first two stages of these diagnoses define criteria for preclinical AD and do not include patients with MCI. The third stage of the NIA-AA criteria includes evidence of cerebral amyloidosis (via CSF or PET studies), evidence of neurodegeneration (changes on structural MRI) and subtle cognitive change not meeting MCI criteria. Stage 4 NIA-AA criteria are the same as those for stage 3, plus evidence of MCI. The NIA-AA criteria differ from the Dubois criteria primarily in the rank ordering of the importance of biomarkers, with CSF or PET scan evidence of cerebral amyloid deposition being regarded as the most definitive biomarker for AD at any stage of the disease.

AD8 QUESTIONNAIRE

1. Problems with judgment (e.g. problems making decisions, bad financial decisions, problems with thinking)
2. Less interest in hobbies/activities
3. Repeating the same things over and over (questions, stories, or statements)
4. Trouble learning how to use a tool, appliance, or gadget (e.g. VCR, computer, microwave, remote control)
5. Forgetting correct month or year
6. Trouble handling complicated financial affairs (e.g. balancing check book, income taxes, paying bills)
7. Trouble remembering appointments
8. Problems with thinking and/or memory

MCI-AD CRITERIA

1. A concern about a change in cognition from a previous level, identified by the patient, an informant, or a skilled clinician.
2. Impairment in one or more cognitive domains. Performance considered to be lower than would be expected, considering the patient's age and education (impairment is typically 1–1.5 standard deviations below the mean of the individual, adjusted for age and education). Impairments may be present in more than one domain and may be amnestic or non-amnestic.
3. Preservation of independence in functional abilities. This criterion allows mild problems with complex tasks to be present, as long as independence of functions, such as paying bills, preparing meals or shopping, is maintained, albeit with minimal aids and assistance.
4. Not demented. The cognitive changes should be sufficiently mild that there is no evidence of impairment in social or occupational function.

Based on much of the afore-mentioned information and guidelines for a diagnosis of AD in a predementia stage, two proposals have been put forth for diagnosis of dementia in an MCI stage. The Dubois criteria for "prodromal AD" published in 2007 require the patient to have amnestic MCI, along with a positive biomarker for AD (e.g. medial temporal atrophy on

VaMCI

Historically, the role of vascular damage in cognitive disorders was well recognized by 19th-century clinicians. However, criteria for MCI and dementia related to vascular disease have been influenced by the concepts used to develop criteria for Alzheimer disease. As a result, a memory disorder has been required in addition to other cognitive deficits for the diagnosis of vascular dementia. Moreover, strokes were thought to be the principal cause of what is now termed vascular dementia (VaD) but was initially known as multiinfarct dementia. The importance of the location of vascular lesions led to the concept of single "strategic" infarcts as a cause of cognitive impairment. Other types of vascular lesions, including white matter hyperintensities on MRI scans, achieved recognition as contributors to progressive cognitive impairment. Recognition that cognitive deficits caused solely by vascular lesions infrequently lead to dementia resulted in the concept of vascular MCI (VaMCI).

The new criteria for VaMCI include four types: amnestic, amnestic plus other domains, non-amnestic single domain, and non-amnestic multiple domains. To decrease the chances of misclassification of VaMCI, at least four cognitive domains must be tested, including memory, visuospatial function, executive function/attention, and language. The criteria for probable and possible VaMCI are similar to those for VaD mentioned above, except that the degree of impairment in instrumental activities of daily living cannot be more than mildly impaired (American Heart Association/American Stroke Association). A category of unstable VaMCI is reserved for patients whose symptoms recede and who return to normal. Possible VaD (or VaMCI) is similar to Probable VaD/VaMCI, but allows for uncertainty in any of the following: temporal relationship between vascular event and cognitive dysfunction, insufficient imaging data, or evidence of a co-existing neurodegenerative cause.

AMERICAN HEART ASSOCIATION CRITERIA FOR PROBABLE VaD

1. Impairment in at least two cognitive domains (not necessarily including memory).
2. A temporal relationship between the vascular insult and cognitive consequences, OR the vascular damage is consistent with the extent or pattern of the cognitive deficit.
3. Functional decline that is not limited to motor or sensory sequelae of a stroke.
4. No history of gradual cognitive decline before the stroke or vascular injury occurred.

Reversible causes of MCI and VaMCI require vigilance on the part of the clinician. Hypothyroidism, cobalamin deficiency (vitamin B12), and metabolic disturbances related to chronic or acute medical conditions such as renal insufficiency, liver failure, and anemia should all be ruled out by sending appropriate blood work. A number of vascular conditions can lead to potentially reversible causes of cognitive impairment. Congestive heart failure leads to reduced brain perfusion, especially as the ejection fraction drops below 20%, and medical therapy as well as heart transplantation can lead to improved cognition. Similarly, large vessel occlusions can lead to cognitive impairment that is potentially reversible. For example, some patients with bilateral carotid occlusions who undergo extracranial to intracranial bypass have dramatic improvements in cognition. However, it is also important to note that patients with moderately advanced AD pathology do not benefit from carotid endarterectomy, so patients need to be carefully selected on a case-by-case basis for these types of procedures.

Differential diagnosis of etiological subtypes of mild cognitive impairment

The clinical features of etiological subtypes of MCI would be expected to be similar to those of the corresponding dementia subtype, with the caveat that not all the typical features of each etiological subtype are likely to be manifest in the MCI stage. For example, one of the distinguishing clinical features used for diagnosing AD is gradually progressive impairment in recent as opposed to remote memory. This feature is generally most apparent in the earlier phases of AD and becomes less distinct in the later stages of the disease. Similarly, visual hallucinations, which are a characteristic symptom of LBD in the dementia stage, are relatively unusual in the MCI stage of the disease. The distinguishing clinical features of each of the major etiological subtypes of MCI are listed in Table 6.2 and Figure 6.2.

Table 6.2 Diagnosis of etiological subtypes of MCI syndromes

Etiological subtypes	Common MCI subtype	Important clinical features	MRI features	Amyloid status (CSF/PET)
Alzheimer's disease	Amnestic	Slowly progressive recent memory impairment	Medial temporal atrophy (MTA)	>60% positive
Lewy body disease	Non-amnestic	REM-BD; attentional deficits and fluctuation, visual hallucinations, tremor, falls rigidity and gait disorder	Little or no MTA, enlarged lateral and third ventricles	Positive if associated with AD pathology
FTLD	Amnestic/non-amnestic	Aphasia, apathy, disinhibition, poor judgment, disproportionate functional impairment	Frontal, lateral temporal and parietal atrophy, asymmetry ++	Negative in over 60%
Vascular cognitive impairment	Non-amnestic	Sudden onset, H/O stroke, focal signs, gait disorder	Evidence of infarcts (commonly in deep gray matter), white matter hyperintensities ++	Positive only if associated with AD pathology
Systemic illness and medication effects	Non-amnestic	Weight loss, fatigue, sleep disorder, headache	Normal	Negative in over 60%
Psychiatric illness	Amnestic	Anxiety, depression, sleep disorder, little or no functional impairment	Normal	Negative in over 60%

AD, Alzheimer's disease; CSF, cerebrospinal fluid; FTLD, frontotemporal lobe degeneration; H/O, history of; MCI, mild cognitive impairment; MRI, magnetic resonance imaging; PET, positron emission tomography; REM-BD, REM-BD, rapid eye movement sleep behavior disorder.

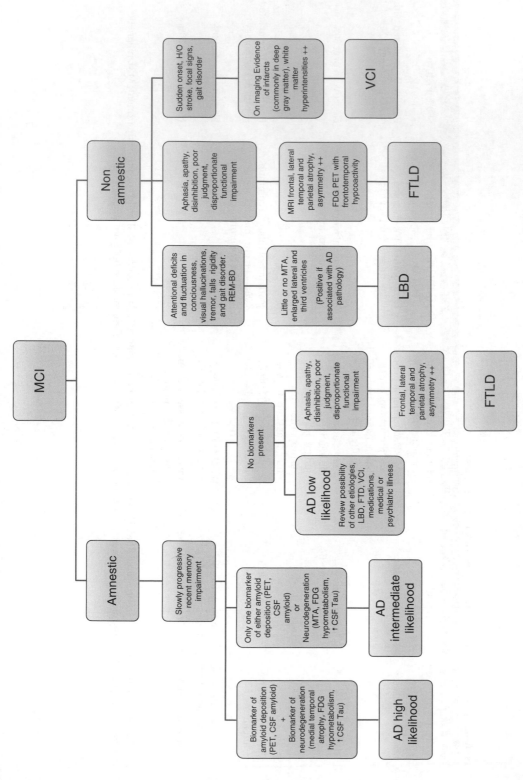

Figure 6.2 MCI diagnostic algorithm. AD, Alzheimer's disease; CSF, cerebrospinal fluid; PET, positron emission tomography; FDG, fluoro-2-deoxy-D-glucose; FTD, frontotemporal dementia; FTLD, frontotemporal lobe degeneration; H/O, history of; LBD, Lewy body dementia; MCI, mild cognitive impairment; MTA, medial temporal atrophy; REM-BD, rapid eye movement sleep behavior disorder; VCI, vascular cognitive impairment.

Psychiatric aspects of mild cognitive impairment

It has been well established that neuropsychiatric symptoms are common and persistent features of Alzheimer's disease. In fact, these symptoms have an estimated prevalence of 50–80% and are typically seen in the later stages of the disorder. Those patients who suffer from psychiatric syndromes as a consequence of degenerative cognitive disorders demonstrate worse functionality and increased caregiver burden. In addition, there is a growing recognition that depression, apathy, agitation, and anxiety may actually be observed in the early stages of MCI and may be seen in approximately 30% of such patients. Patients presenting with four or more neuropsychiatric symptoms are more likely to be diagnosed with aMCI and, conversely, patients diagnosed with aMCI are more likely to exhibit depressive symptoms than other symptoms and have an increased risk of developing dementia.

The relationship between depression and dementia is a complex one, with the results of some studies suggesting that depression may often be a prodrome to AD, whereas other studies suggest that impaired attention and executive function are associated with geriatric depression and that these deficits may persist even after successful treatment of depression. Subjects with MCI who had prominent deficits in executive functioning were found to have greater severity of depression. In addition to models depicting "depression as prodrome" and "depression as a consequence" of neurodegeneration, other models suggest that depression may actually be an important risk factor for the development of Alzheimer's disease. Further complicating the picture is the fact that patients with minor depression or dysthymia may have symptoms that may be associated with stress and emotional strain due to having impaired cognition. Given the heterogeneity of MCI, depression may reflect an underlying etiology other than AD, such as cerebrovascular or frontotemporal neurodegenerative disease, which may disrupt frontostriatal pathways, leading to symptoms of a mood disorder, or frontal lobe symptoms such as apathy or disinhibition.

★ TIPS AND TRICKS

Apathy can be frequently confused with depression in patients with MCI. In general, apathy is much less responsive to pharmacological interventions compared to depression.

Making the diagnosis of depression in MCI patients can be challenging for the clinician. It is not uncommon for older adults with depression to present with irritability, anxiety, and apathy rather than complaining of sadness or depressed mood. Although it is important that clinicians be aware that memory complaints may be symptomatic of underlying depression, it is important, especially for psychiatrists, to be aware that depressive symptoms in an individual who has demonstrable amnestic deficits often suggest an early form of dementia. Apathy is also a common psychiatric symptom in both MCI and AD and can by itself cause significant distress in family members and caregivers. It may also cause significant dysfunction in patients and may prevent them from seeking necessary medical treatment and they may become non-compliant with their medical regimens. Apathy as a clinical syndrome is also often mistaken for the signs and symptoms of depression in that both conditions share certain characteristics, such as lack of interest and motivation. What is often distinct about depression is dysphoric mood or irritability. In addition, patients with depression also frequently suffer from feelings of hopelessness, guilt, anxiety, worthlessness, and preoccupation with death.

Although hallucinations and delusions are frequently observed in AD, these symptoms are relatively uncommon in patients with MCI. Visual hallucinations, in concert with rapid eye movement (REM) sleep behavior disorder, in a patient presenting with MCI should alert clinicians to the possibility of early Lewy body disease.

Ethical considerations of early diagnosis of predementia states

The relatively modest attendant benefits of currently available treatments must be balanced against the cost of the evaluations and medical treatments. An earlier diagnosis of AD allows important medical, social, and financial management decisions to be made sooner by the patient and family members. However, a certain proportion of patients and their families may regard the diagnosis of MCI as an earlier version of a progressive dementing condition, as threatening, intrusive and unwelcome, regardless of any potential benefits of early intervention. Misclassification and mislabeling of individuals who are in fact disease free is also more likely when diagnosis is attempted at an earlier stage of a disease.

The ultimate decision to proceed with making an earlier diagnosis of AD in a patient who does not meet criteria for dementia should be determined by the patient and caregiver with the advice of the referring physician. The positive and negative medical, social, and economic considerations in each case with MCI should be individualized before launching into a potentially expensive clinical evaluation.

If it is decided to proceed with a diagnostic evaluation, it will be important to individualize how the diagnosis is to be conveyed to the patent and family members who are authorized to receive the diagnosis. While patients have the right to obtain the diagnosis made by a physician, the physician should not feel obliged to force the diagnosis on the patient. In this respect, the physician must try to exercise judgment about how much the patient wants to know and determine how best to convey that information, such that it maximizes the likelihood of the best outcomes for patient and family. Consideration should be given to the impact the diagnosis may have on the psychological and emotional state of the patient and family, the patient's employment, coverage by various insurance companies, including long-term care and life insurance, as well as on the potential for social isolation of patient and family members. In conjunction with conveying the diagnosis of a progressively dementing disorder, the goal of the physician should be to identify clearly in what situations the patient's cognitive and functional deficits pose a substantial risk for the patient and for others (e.g. driving, investing money, hunting). At the same time, the physician should try and avoid imposing unnecessary curtailment of the patient's activities and employment, or ability to make choices and interact socially.

Predictors of rate of progression of mild cognitive impairment to dementia

The rate of progression from MCI to a dementia state is used to provide an index of the underlying neuropathological process in a particular subject group. In clinical settings, the rate of progression from amnestic MCI to dementia is generally 10–15% per year. As might be expected, the prevalence rates of MCI and the rates of progression to dementia among subjects diagnosed in a community setting appear to be considerably lower than for subjects seen in a clinic setting. Other well-established predictors are the severity and duration of cognitive (especially memory) impairment, the severity of medial temporal atrophy and white matter hyperintensities on MRI, and severity of neocortical hypometabolism on FDG-PET. The presence of extrapyramidal signs, vascular risk factors, and elevated levels of tau protein in cerebrospinal fluid are all associated with greater risk for progressing to dementia, and combinations of these risk factors are found to be additive in some studies, increasing the risk 5–12-fold. Depression, especially in the presence of co-morbid anxiety, predicts progression to dementia, although the presence of neither depression nor anxiety has been found to predict the likelihood of reversion to a normal cognitive state among those with MCI.

The APOE gene has been found to be the most potent genetic risk factor for sporadically occurring AD; nevertheless, it is not clear whether the APOE 4 allele accelerates the rate of progression from MCI to AD. The risk for conversion to dementia appears to be most evident among the youngest MCI subjects who are APOE 4 genotype carriers. The Predementia Alzheimer's Disease Scale (PAS) combines demographic, cognitive, and biomarker profiles and the resulting score has been shown to be associated with an increased risk of progression from normal cognition to MCI. The best predictors of the progression from MCI to AD in the PAS are age, memory scores, presence of hypertension, APOE 4 genotype, and hippocampal atrophy.

⚗ SCIENCE REVISITED

The Predementia Alzheimer's Disease Scale (PAS) aims to identify subjects with mild cognitive impairments (or cognitive impairment no dementia) who are in the preclinical stage of AD. The PAS consists of six items: age, MMSE score, functional impairment, cognitive test performance, apolipoprotein E (apoE) genotype, and medial temporal lobe (MTL) atrophy. Each variable can be scored on a 3- or 4-point scale and the sum score determines the risk for AD. It has been shown that a PAS score >=6 is associated with a high risk for subsequent AD, a score of 5 with a borderline risk and a score <=4 with a low risk for AD. The PAS score was shown to correlate with the level of phospho-tau and beta-amyloid 1-42 in cerebrospinal fluid, suggesting that the PAS indeed reflects AD pathology[8].

Treatment of mild cognitive impairment

Several treatment trials are ongoing, with the goal of slowing or reversing the course of cognitive and functional decline among MCI subjects, including the use of gamma-secretase inhibitors to influence amyloid deposition rates and vaccines to remove amyloid from the brain. Thus far no treatment trials have successfully slowed progression from MCI to dementia although medications currently approved for the treatment of AD and other dementias, such as donepezil, rivastigmine, and galantamine, are often used for treating MCI patients. Although trials with these medications have not been found to decrease the rate of progression in longer term studies (e.g. 3 years), in the first 12 months donepezil was found to reduce the risk of progressing to AD and among APOE 4 carriers a small but significant benefit was found at 3 years. These results were not considered strong enough to recommend donepezil as a treatment for MCI patients, but provide a rationale for considering donepezil as an option at the MCI stage.

Treatment of VaMCI should be determined by appropriate management of the underlying vascular disease. Aggressive risk factor control has the potential to limit further damage and prevent progression of cognitive decline. Those with heart failure and large vessel occlusions may benefit from medical and surgical options as well, as noted above. In the case of LBD, it has anecdotally been reported that in the dementia stage there is often a very encouraging cognitive response to treatment with cholinesterase inhibitors. Although no data are yet available on treatment of MCI-LBD with cholinesterase inhibitors, it may be expected that response to these agents should be similar to that seen in LBD cases who have dementia. Treatment of MCI-FTLD, as is the case for FTLD in the dementia stage, is directed mainly to the associated behavioral and psychiatric disturbances (see below). Patients with LBD tend to respond adversely to antipsychotic medications, which may accelerate progression to dementia among MCI-LBD patients.

> ### ✋ CAUTION
>
> Avoid using antipsychotics with high risk of extrapyramidal side-effects (haloperidol, risperidone) in patients who have symptoms suggestive of Lewy body disease. Quetiapine, which has less potential for extrapyramidal side-effects, would be a better option.

There are minimal data on the treatment of psychiatric symptoms in MCI; however, the treatment benefit in AD has been documented to improve psychiatric symptoms and patients' functional abilities. Therefore, it would appear prudent to treat those psychiatric symptoms that are distressing to patients. Antidepressant treatments such as selective serotonin reuptake inhibitors (SSRIs) are indicated as first line in the treatment of depression in MCI. Medications with anticholinergic side-effects such as tricyclic antidepressants should be avoided as they might exacerbate cognitive symptoms. Antipsychotics are frequently used in the treatment of psychosis, particularly early diffuse Lewy body disease; however, they should be used with extreme caution due to the risk of increased mortality when used in cognitively impaired elderly, and should be avoided when treating anxiety or insomnia. Apathy syndromes can be treated with methylphenidate and activating antidepressants, such as bupropion, although there is no conclusive evidence that they work.

Non-pharmacological approaches to MCI and early dementia may have a useful and perhaps more effective role in preventing progression of aMCI to dementia. A well-controlled clinical trial of physical exercise and cognitive function among elderly normal subjects and those with MCI suggests that exercise may enhance cognition among these subjects. Cognitive rehabilitative procedures, including face-name association and spaced retrieval, can improve cognitive function and improve functional skills, using motor and procedural learning techniques and paradigms that enhance the speed of cognitive processing. All these techniques make use of the family member as a therapy extender and also employ memory notebooks as compensatory strategies.

Prevention of mild cognitive impairment among at-risk cognitively normal elderly people

The most important lessons learned for prevention of coronary artery disease are also applicable for prevention of cognitive impairment. These measures include those relating to lifestyle changes and scrupulous management of all medical risk factors for vascular disease. In addition, it is important to avoid the chronic use of medications, commonly used in the elderly, that are anticholinergic or sedative (such as benzodiazepines), and it is also important to avoid excessive consumption of alcohol. Finally, certain supplements and prescription medications have the potential for reducing the risk of late-life cognitive decline.

Lifestyle changes

These include:

- cessation of smoking
- dietary changes to emphasize weight loss among those above ideal weight, a low intake of carbohydrate and fats, a high intake of proteins, vegetable, fruit, spices and nuts (especially those that provide high antioxidant and antiinflammatory benefit), moderate alcohol and caffeine consumption
- regular aerobic exercises (about 45 min every day, 7 days a week, including going to the gym, walking, bicycling, jogging and dancing)
- stress-free social interactions, hobbies (such as gardening, painting, reading for pleasure, listening to music) and mental stimulation in cultural and intellectual activities.

Management of medical risk factors

Relevant medical conditions that should be detected as early as possible and managed optimally include treatment of hypertension, diabetes mellitus, coronary artery disease and arrhythmias, elevated cholesterol and lipids, peripheral vascular disease, carotid artery disease, sleep apnea and chronic lung diseases, chronic renal disease, medication, drug and alcohol abuse.

The rate of cognitive decline in longitudinal studies is well known to be associated positively with the systolic and diastolic blood pressure, as well as with elevated serum cholesterol levels. Type 2 diabetes mellitus has been strongly associated with an increased risk of cognitive impairment and AD. In one study 43% of dementia risk was attributable to diabetes mellitus, stroke or the combination. High insulin levels, seen in type 2 diabetes mellitus, may convey a specific risk for brain amyloid deposition and future risk for developing AD.

Avoidance of chronic use of certain prescription medications

Anticholinergic medications (both prescription and over the counter) are used very commonly for the treatment of various conditions in the elderly, in particular. These include medications for the treatment of insomnia (especially diphenhydramine and amytriptiline), incontinence, dizziness and vertigo (especially meclizine), allergies and chronic itching, depression, gastrointestinal spasms, and hyperacidity.

Use of supplements and prescription medications

Certain supplements and medications may reduce the risk of developing dementing diseases, such as AD, as well as the rate of progression, especially in the earliest stages. Epidemiological evidence and individual clinical trials suggest that factors identified for lowering the risk of chronic diseases such as stroke, diabetes, and vascular diseases also reduce risk for AD. Most notable among these are vitamins C and B12, pyridoxine and other B vitamins, and omega 3 fatty acids, most conveniently obtained in fish oil supplements. There are some preliminary data suggesting that certain antihypertensive medications (angiotensin converting enzyme inhibitors and angiotensin receptor blockers) as well as statin medications may be particularly useful for prevention of cardiovascular and neurodegenerative disease, but the data are not strong enough to warrant specific treatment recommendations at this time.

References

[1] Petersen RC, Smith GE, Waring S, et al. Mild cognitive impairment: clinical characterization and outcome. *Arch Neurol* 1999; **56**: 303–8.

[2] Petersen RC, Morris JC. Clinical features. In: Petersen RC (ed) *Mild Cognitive Impairment: Aging to Alzheimer's Disease*. New York: Oxford University Press, 2003, pp15–39.

[3] Grundman M, Petersen RC, Ferris S, et al. Mild cognitive impairment can be distinguished from Alzheimer disease and normal aging for clinical trials. *Arch Neurol* 2004; **61**: 59–66.

[4] Petersen RC, Stevens JC, Ganguli M, et al. Practice parameter: early detection of dementia: mild cognitive impairment (an evidence-based review). Report of the Quality Standards Subcommittee of the American Academy of Neurology. Neurology 2001; **56**: 1133–42.

[5]   Duara R, Loewenstein DA, Potter E, et al. Medial temporal lobe atrophy on MRI scans and the diagnosis of Alzheimer's disease. *Neurology* 2008; **71**: 1986–92.

[6]   Urs R, Potter E, Barker W, et al. Visual rating system (VRS) for assessing magnetic resonance images (MRIs): a tool in the diagnosis of MCI and Alzheimer's disease. *J Comput Assist Tomogr* 2009; **33**(1): 73–8.

[7]   Dubois B, Feldman H, Jacova C, et al. Research criteria for the diagnosis of Alzheimer's disease: revising the NINCDS-ADRDA criteria. *Lancet Neurol* 2007; **6**: 734–46.

[8]   Visser P, Scheltens P, Verhey F. Diagnostic accuracy of the Predementia AD Scale (PAS) in cognitively mildly impaired subjects. *J Neurol* 2002; **249**: 312–19.

Further reading

Barker WW, Luis C, Kashuba A, et al. Relative frequencies of Alzheimer disease, Lewy body, vascular and frontotemporal dementia, and hippocampal sclerosis in the state of Florida brain bank. *Alzheimer's Dis Assoc Disord* 2002; **16**: 203–12.

Braak H, Braak E. Diagnostic criteria for neuropathological assessment of Alzheimer's disease. *Neurobiol Aging* 1997; **18**(Suppl): S85–S88.

Ganguli M, Dodge H, Shen C, DeKosky S. Mild cognitive impairment amnestic type: an epidemiologic study. *Neurology* 2004; **63**: 115–21.

Farlow MR. Treatment of mild cognitive impairment (MCI). *Curr Alzheimer Res* 2009; **6**: 362–7.

Galvin JE, Powlishta K, Wilkins K, et al. Predictors of preclinical Alzheimer disease and dementia: a clinicopathologic study. *Arch Neurol* 2005; **62**: 758–65.

Galvin JE, Roe CM, Coats M, Morris J. Patient's rating of cognitive ability: using the AD8, a brief informant interview, as a self-rating tool to detect dementia. *Arch Neurol* 2007; **64**: 725–30.

Gorelick PB, Scuteri A, Black SE, et al. Vascular contributions to cognitive impairment and dementia: a statement for healthcare professionals from the American Heart Association/American Stroke Association. *Stroke* 2011; **42**: 2672–713.

Jack CR Jr, Knopman DS, Jagust W, et al. Hypothetical model of dynamic biomarkers of the Alzheimer's pathological cascade. *Lancet Neurol* 2010; **9**: 119–28.

Loewenstein DA, Barker WW, Harwood DG, et al. Utility of a modified mini-mental state examination with extended delayed recall in screening for mild cognitive impairment and dementia among community dwelling elders. *Int J Geriatr Psychiatry* 2000; **15**: 434– 40.

7

After the Diagnosis: Continuing Neurological Care of the Outpatient with Dementia

Anne M. Lipton

Diplomate in Neurology, American Board of Psychiatry and Neurology, Canada

Introduction: from diagnosis to care

It's not usually difficult to make a diagnosis of *severe* dementia of unspecified type, but a vague diagnosis made at this late stage does not allow for the early and appropriate intervention, planning, and support that patients and families deserve. Unfortunately, dementia goes undiagnosed in 50% or more of individuals in the mild-to-moderate stages of this disease. Reviewing the previous chapter should have heightened your awareness and clinical acumen regarding dementia and help you to make – and not to miss – this diagnosis. Patients with dementia often possess poor insight into their problems, but this symptom should not be contagious to doctors!

Diagnosing a *specific* type of dementia (i.e. rather than making a diagnosis of generic dementia/ dementia, not otherwise specified or calling all dementia Alzheimer's disease) represents the true challenge for physicians. Remember: *Alzheimer's is not the only dementia*.

Such specificity guides treatment and prognostication, an issue families commonly raise ("How long does he have, doc?") upon hearing a diagnosis of dementia. It therefore behooves a doctor to broach the subject of prognosis, even if not raised by the family, as it may be an unspoken question. (Patients usually don't ask this question, perhaps due to poor insight and/or difficulty with complex information processing.) The same applies to genetics. A sensible rule is to address questions of prognosis and heredity to at least some degree, even if not specifically asked. (Both of these topics will be covered in more detail later in this chapter.)

Specificity of diagnosis guides management most during the beginning and middle stages of dementia. Such precision may become less essential as dementia advances and options for planning and interventions diminish. That is to say, all dementias start differently but tend to go towards the same endpoint. Although care strategies may become more restricted as dementia progresses, choices remain consequential throughout. A physician plays a crucial role in educating families (or other medical decision makers) about available options, including alternatives to futile and potentially harmful treatments (see Chapter 9).

Neurologists should strive for a timely and specific diagnosis, since different dementia subtypes may warrant different treatments. The remainder of this chapter focuses mainly on shared principles of compassionate neurological care for patients with dementia. More extensive information about tailored approaches for diverse types of dementia may be found in a variety of web-based and print sources (see Further Reading). Especially when faced with a dementia type with which you lack familiarity, consult these resources and/or a dementia specialist, such as a behavioral neurologist or geriatric psychiatrist. Given the shortage of practitioners in these specialties, a general psychiatrist or geriatrician may meet your needs and those of your patient.

Dementia, First Edition. Edited by Joseph F. Quinn.
© 2014 John Wiley & Sons, Ltd. Published 2014 by John Wiley & Sons, Ltd.

What is the role for the neurologist after diagnosis?

Many neurologists continue to take the "diagnose and adios" approach to dementia patients, leaving the follow-up care to primary care providers. In the absence of interventions requiring the particular knowledge or skills of a specialist, this is a defensible practice at the present time. However, many patients and families prefer periodic follow-up with a specialist to review their status, their medications, and overall care plans. This chapter is intended to provide some practical guidance for neurologists who elect to provide this type of continuing care for dementia patients. The little bit of evidence that exists on the subject indicates that dementia care is improved by the continuing care of specialists, whether neurologists or geriatricians.

The delineation of treatment goals may help justify the participation of neurologists in dementia care. Treatment goals change during the course of the disease, from preservation of function in early stages, to management of behavioral problems in middle stages, to palliative care in later stages, but there is a potential role for neurologists at each of these stages (Table 7.1). This chapter serves as a guide to management across all stages, with other chapters dedicated to the details of pharmacological management of behavior problems and palliative care in later stages.

Table 7.1 Examples of stage-specific treatment management of dementia

Stage	Treatment goals	Specific strategies
Mild	Maintaining function	Cholinesterase inhibitors Treatment of co-morbidities (e.g. vascular risk factors, depression) Optimize nutrition, exercise Caregiver education
Moderate	Manage behavioral problems Delay residential care	Simplify environment Adopt consistent routine Addition of memantine Judicious use of psychotropic meds Caregiver support
Severe	Patient comfort	Support caregiver in transition to residential care Hospice referral

Partnering in dementia care

Patients with dementia tend to have poor insight even in the early stages of this disease. Therefore, most will not bring up their cognitive or behavioral issues independently. Typically, a family member accompanies (or brings, sometimes with strong encouragement) a loved one with "memory problems" or suspected dementia for evaluation. However, you may see a patient for a different neurological complaint and note problems indicative of dementia. This warrants an attempt to include family members (or other responsible party) at subsequent visits.

A patient with dementia should have a medical partner to attend all doctors' visits. In practice, this is often a family member. However, some patients may have a friend, partner, neighbor, professional caregiver, or other who plays this role. (Therefore, note that reference and recommendations in this chapter for the medical and supportive role of a "family member" or "family caregiver" may apply to another individual so involved.) Ideally, this person would be the designated Medical Power of Attorney (MPOA), either acting in this role currently or a durable MPOA upon patient's incapacity, and able to attend all doctors' visits. In practice, sometimes different family members rotate responsibility for attending doctors' visits. Having one family member act as "gatekeeper" or point person to coordinate all of a patient's medical care works well. At the very least, if multiple family members rotate, recommend that one family member works with one physician and reports updates to this point person. The person who has durable or active MPOA should be encouraged to attend visits since this person should be well acquainted with the patient's care, as he or she is making medical decisions on the patient's behalf (or will be doing so in the future). For example, it becomes cumbersome to discuss and contemplate relatively straightforward and routine matters such as side-effects of medication, let alone handle crisis management, if a MPOA is not present at a follow-up appointment. For a patient who has capacity, a frank discussion should be undertaken regarding the clear advantages of designating someone as durable MPOA who can be well acquainted with the patient's medical wishes, history, treatment, and team. For those patients who no longer have capacity, the person acting as MPOA should be involved via telephone or other communication at appointments, regarding treatment decisions, etc. Preferably, the same person can attend all doctors' visits and act as MPOA, if needs be. Visits should be scheduled when the patient and at least one family member (or other medical partner) can attend together.

In all cases, Health Insurance Portability and Accountability Act (HIPPA) and other requirements for protecting private health information (PHI) should be followed, such as obtaining patient consent to discuss PHI with relevant parties. It is important to have HIPPA forms signed by a person capable of doing so. A patient with incapacity due to dementia or other reasons cannot legally agree or refuse consent. Patients who agree that someone may accompany them during doctors' visits are granting permission for discussion of private health information with that person, but it is best to document this consent. Chapter 10 discusses these issues in further detail.

Diagnostic considerations specific to dementia

It is not a good idea to inform patients of a dementia diagnosis or prescribe an antidementia medication without a companion for support, as well as to provide information for diagnosis, remember medication and other information discussed, and advocate in terms of asking questions and monitoring progress until the next visit.

If patients forget their dementia diagnosis, just let them. Some patients may lack awareness of the full extent and consequences of their dementia. Use memory loss to advantage and let ignorance be bliss. Advise families of this as well. Testing outside the clinic should also be avoided to prevent patient anxiety – and practice effect!

Families and other carers should, of course, step in to protect patient safety, but this need not include repeatedly reminding patients with dementia of their diagnosis. In dementia, correction, criticism, and reprimands should generally be avoided. This is a crucial principle in the day-to-day care of patients with dementia: *Avoid conflict and go with the flow.*

Using simpler terms – or even better, simply providing reassurance – usually trumps more complex clinical terms for most people, patients and caregivers alike. The bottom line is that short, simple explanations usually work well for patients with dementia. Answering the same query repeatedly is annoying at best. Having a short answer, especially writing it down, or having a visual reminder (such as a calendar) usually works best. This is another important principle that resonates throughout dementia care: *Show, don't tell.*

> ⭐ **TIPS AND TRICKS**
>
> Each patient with dementia should have a medical partner (often a family member or other close individual) to attend doctors' visits, provide medication list and other updates, and help advocate for patient interests.

Families (and others) can provide vital information on a patient's symptoms and clinical course. However, they may find it hard to discuss problems such as excessive alcohol intake, hallucinations, inappropriate social behaviors (e.g. disrobing in public), unsafe driving, and difficulty managing finances, particularly in the presence of the patient. When evaluating someone with anosognosia (a lack of awareness into one's own problems), probing almost any issue may be tricky.

Ask family members or other medical partners to jot down two or three of their major concerns on *one* sheet of paper and bring it to the visit. They might even hand this page discreetly to check-in staff to avoid having to give it directly to you in front of the patient. Such a note allows you to "hear" family concerns and garner necessary information about the patient's mental status, behavior, and function, while minimizing the potential for embarrassing or even explosive situations.

> ★ **TIPS AND TRICKS**
>
> Encourage families to put concerns in writing.

Family conferences

If it is difficult to formulate or execute a plan of care in a patient's presence due to that individual's cognitive and/or behavioral condition, it may be necessary to conduct a family conference without the patient (e.g., a patient who becomes highly agitated with any discussion or paces for the entire visit). Such sessions may be conducted so long as HIPPA and other regulations protecting a patient's PHI are honored (e.g. with consent of the MPOA if a patient lacks capacity for medical decision making). Medicare and other insurance typically does *not* cover the cost of such meetings. Families should be informed upfront of any fees. These conferences may work well for families with multiple members, particularly those who may not attend doctors' visits routinely and/or live out of town but wish to meet and ask questions directly of the doctor and out of earshot of the patient.

Medications

Medication list and supervision

Any of us can forget a medication. It makes little sense to prescribe medication for memory and similar problems without a mechanism to monitor if such remedies are taken correctly. (In fact, it might be quite harmful to do so.)

Request that both patient and family member work together to assemble a list of the patient's medications and that each should carry this (either on a card in a wallet or as a list in a smartphone). This ensures availability in case of an emergency and for all doctors' visits, facilitating review of medications and potential interactions, risks, and benefits. Three requirements that should be met prior to prescribing medications for a patient with dementia are a medication list, a pillbox (or similar system), and supervision (or out-and-out administration) by a responsible family member or professional.

Use of a weekly pillbox (with a number of daily slots commensurate with the maximum daily frequency of any medication) provides a convenient mechanism for a family member. A relative (or other caregiver) can help a patient fill such a device, which also allows the opportunity to refill medications before they run out as well as to check for missed dosages (which, if identified, indicate a need for increased supervision and assistance with medications). Such a pillbox should be located somewhere prominently (e.g. on a kitchen table) and linked to another habit (such as eating breakfast). Someone who lives with a patient might use their own pillbox for any vitamins or medications to lend moral support to the patient and help make it a part of the household routine.

Recommend that family members partner with patients or assume full responsibility for prescription refills. Older patients, in particular, may accept the assistance of their adult children, when a doctor recommends and/or the grown children volunteer to order these online for parents who are not as adept on the computer, particularly due to the cost savings that this may provide.

> ★ **TIPS AND TRICKS**
>
> A list of medications and a plan to ensure that a patient doesn't forget to take them are prerequisites for prescribing drugs for memory loss or similar symptoms. A pillbox which a family member or other caregiver helps fill and check represents a good starting point. Missed doses indicate a need for additional supervision and assistance (i.e. beyond use of a pillbox). Family caregivers should also assist in obtaining prescription refills.

Prescribing considerations

Out with the bad, in with the good

Review current medications, especially before initiating any new ones. Agents that may adversely affect memory and other aspects of cognition should be minimized. Similarly, a patient with dementia may be exquisitely sensitized to amnestic and other adverse effects of alcohol, and its use may need to be reduced or altogether avoided.

Start low and go slow – but keep going

This is the mantra of behavioral and geriatric neurology. While a careful initial titration is important, it is also crucial to *keep going* to achieve an effective dose and maintain this for enough time to give the drug a fair trial. This is particularly the case in dementia since available medications are by no means curative and, at best, only slow the inexorable declines in cognition, behavior, and function.

Antidementia medications

Practical tips are offered for use of the products described herein. Full labeling information should be consulted before prescribing these or any medications.

While dementia is primarily irreversible and incurable, most dementia *is* treatable to some extent. The main agents used are sometimes called cognitive enhancers, but the term antidementia medications better reflects their more widespread effects, including with regard to behavior and function. (The following chapter addresses the use of medications for behavioral issues in dementia.)

Only two major classes of medication have FDA approval for treatment of dementia (and then only specific types and stages of dementia, as discussed below). These are the cholinesterase inhibitors and the N-methyl-D-aspartate (NMDA) antagonist memantine.

Cholinesterase inhibitors (CIs)

These include donepezil, galantamine, and rivastigmine. Alzheimer's disease (AD) is associated with loss of cholinergic neurons and reduction in available acetylcholine. These drugs act to reduce the reuptake of this neurotransmitter, increasing the availability of acetylcholine. Common side-effects are gastrointestinal (GI), such as nausea and diarrhea. Bradycardia and syncope represent less common but serious adverse effects. Insomnia and nightmares are also

possible, so, for those agents that are administered once a day, this author prefers prescribing these off-label in the morning (after breakfast) to help minimize the risk of these symptoms.

Donepezil

This drug is approved for all stages of AD and available in tablets in a variety of dosage. The orally disintegrating tablet (ODT) form may be useful for patients with dysphagia or other difficulty taking pills. The dosage titrations should be attempted only after at least 4 weeks on a given dose (e.g. 5 mg daily × 28 days, then 10 mg daily). As noted above, this author prefers prescribing these off-label in the morning (after breakfast) to help minimize the risk of GI symptoms and sleep disturbance.

Galantamine

This medication is approved for mild-to-moderate stage AD and is available in tablets and oral solution dosed twice a day and extended-release capsules administered daily. The dosage titrations should be attempted only after at least 4 weeks on a given dose As noted above, this author prefers prescribing these off-label in the morning (after breakfast) to help minimize the risk of GI symptoms and sleep disturbance.

Rivastigmine

Approved for mild-to-moderate stage AD, this is the only drug also approved for Parkinson's disease dementia. It is also the only CI available as a (daily) patch. Other forms include twice-a-day capsules in a variety of dosages. Dosage titrations should be attempted only after at least 4 weeks on a given dose.

NMDA antagonist

Memantine is a non-competitive NMDA antagonist and the only drug in this class which has an FDA indication for treatment of dementia. It is generally well tolerated, but common adverse effects may include confusion, constipation, dizziness, drowsiness, and headache. It comes in a 28 mg extended-release tablet for once-daily usage as well as 5 and 10 mg tablets FDA approved for twice-daily dosing. However, the half-life of the 5 and 10 mg tablets is 60–100 h, so there appears to be no pharmacological contraindication to off-label once-daily dosing (which is how the same preparation is dosed in Europe and an off-label option this author has utilized in a number of patients. It is particularly useful to switch the entire daily dose to the evening for patients who experience daytime somnolence.)

Combination therapy

This refers to the simultaneous use of a CI and memantine and represents the standard of care for patients with moderate AD. It works well to start one drug and achieve the maximally effective dose on that before starting the other.

Consider the side-effect profile of these products in deciding which one to start first and use this to advantage. For example, many elderly patients experience constipation, so it usually works best to start a CI first, potentially relieving irregularity, before initiating memantine. Alternatively, for a patient with a history of diarrhea, it may be useful to start memantine first. Some patients previously unable to tolerate a CI due to GI side-effects (such as nausea and diarrhea) may be able to do so after starting memantine. In fact, studies of combination therapy show precisely this – that patients taking a CI and memantine together had fewer such GI events than those taking a CI alone. Use of the patch form of a CI should also be considered in patients with such GI symptoms.

> **EVIDENCE AT A GLANCE**
>
> Unbiased systematic reviews (e.g. Cochrane reviews) of CIs and memantine conclude that these symptomatic medicationss are effective in Alzheimer's disease. However, the magnitude of the treatment effects is modest and the clinical importance has been debated.

Managing expectations

Antidementia drugs might result in transient improvements in individual patients, but are generally expected to offer symptomatic treatment. Overall, a picture of slowing cognitive, behavioral, and functional decline may be seen, but improvement should not be expected. Therefore, it is important to manage expectations – your own and those of your patients and their families. That is to say, these drugs should not be stopped merely due to lack of improvement. In the paradigm of dementia care, stabilization of symptoms may be a victory.

> **CASE**
>
> An 82-year-old woman was brought by her two grown daughters to a neurologist's office for evaluation due to dramatic worsening of dementia symptoms over the preceding month. The patient had been diagnosed with Alzheimer's disease by her primary care physician 6 months prior and started on a cholinesterase inhibitor. She had no adverse effects, but the prescribing doctor stopped this medication 6 weeks ago after the daughters reported that their mother's memory had continued to worsen. Over the past month, the patient had developed new symptoms of agitation and irritability, and her daughters wondered whether she needed a new medicine. When the neurologist restarted the patient on the same cholinesterase inhibitor she had taken previously, her mood and behavioral symptoms resolved.

Off-label prescribing

Because no medications are FDA approved for dementia other than AD and Parkinson's disease dementia (PDD), these agents are often prescribed off-label for such dementia types. Caution should be exercised as these medications may not be as effective in dementias other than Alzheimer's and Parkinson's and may have increased or altered risks. For example, CIs tend to ameliorate behavioral problems in AD, but may exacerbate symptoms such as agitation and/or irritability in non-Alzheimer's dementias and even unmask psychosis (hallucinations and/or delusions) in patients who have dementia with Lewy bodies.

Alternative medicine

Since galantamine derives from the snowdrop flower, it may be well suited for patients with a preference for "natural" remedies. (However, its effects have *not* been shown to be any different or superior to other CIs.) Alternative therapies, such as medical foods, other plant-based remedies, vitamins, and other supplements, generally lack convincing evidence of consistent benefit. The Chinese herbal medicine Huperzine A possesses a pharmacological profile similar to cholinesterase inhibitors but failed to show benefit in a randomized controlled trial. And some alternative therapies may do more harm than good. The preponderance of evidence suggests that nutrients ingested as part of a healthy diet probably confer greater benefit than those found in supplements.

> ✋ **CAUTION**
>
> Huperzine A should be avoided in patients taking cholinesterase inhibitors due to a similar, but inefficacious, mechanism of action and overlapping adverse effect profile.

Other medications

Here are a few considerations for the neurologist reviewing medications for a patient with dementia. (See the next chapter for further information regarding agents used to treat mood and behavior symptoms in dementia.)

Anticholinergic agents

The use of these should be minimized for patients with dementia as anticholinergic action corresponds with adverse effects on memory. This class includes many over-the-counter sleep preparations, often with the designation "PM", which contain diphenhydramine. Patients and families should be specifically questioned as to the use of over-the-counter medications and sleep aids, as they often forget to include such information even when asked about medications or creating a medication list.

Many other drugs, such as tricyclic agents, bladder incontinence preparations, and even putatively selective serotonin reuptake inhibitors (SSRIs), possess anticholinergic effects to varying degrees (paroxetine and fluoxetine are among the most anticholinergic of the SSRIs). Careful selection (or avoidance) serves to reduce these effects. For example, rather than prescribing (or continuing) a patient with dementia on amitriptyline or nortriptyline for neuropathy, a different class of agent might minimize adverse effects on memory. Scheduled toileting best addresses bladder incontinence directly due to dementia. Bladder incontinence drugs are best avoided in patients who have to wear incontinence pads and similar products as these medications are probably not enhancing quality of life while adding additional cost and potentially posing adverse effects on cognition.

Antidepressants

As noted above, tricyclic agents and even some SSRIs may have anticholinergic properties and adverse effects on memory. That said, trazodone is helpful for agitation, insomnia, and other behavioral symptoms in dementia (including frontotemporal dementia, FTD). It may be started in doses of 25 mg and prescribed in a standing dose or prn. Doses may be increased in increments of 25 mg, not to exceed a total daily dose of 200 mg. The main side-effect is sedation. Priapism is possible but unlikely, especially in the typical elderly dementia patient.

Benzodiazepines

Due to risks of sedation, falls, and adverse effects on memory, especially for elderly patients, medications in this class (particularly shorter-acting agents, such as alprazolam) should be minimized and avoided, if possible. However, patients who have taken one of these for years have probably developed drug dependence and are unlikely to tolerate weaning.

Sleep aids

Many sleep aids have adverse effects on memory. In some cases, the need for a sleep aid may be obviated by simply changing the timing of dosing preexisting medications, as is the case for the dementia drugs cited above. This is also true for antidepressants. If a patient is sleepy during the day but has insomnia at night, it may serve to switch their antidepressant from morning to evening to see if this will help reduce both symptoms. If a patient is taking a cholinesterase inhibitor at night and experiencing insomnia or nightmares, it may be worth switching this to the morning.

As noted above, benzodiazapines and tricyclic agents should generally be avoided, but trazodone may be useful with a minimum of amnesia. The antidepressant mirtazapine is typically dosed in the evening and also works quite well as a sleep aid. It can be started at a low dose of 7.5 mg qhs and increased as needed by increments of 7.5 mg to address mood, sleep, and anorexia in patients with dementia. At low doses, its side-effects may also include increased appetite and weight gain, both of which may be advantageous for some patients with dementia. Top doses should not exceed 45 mg daily.

Anesthesia and surgery

Anesthesia and surgery are probably not good for the brain, particularly one affected by dementing illness. Some of these effects may not be permanent, but avoidance is probably best. Therefore, elective surgeries should be avoided and only the most necessary of surgeries performed (namely, those that confer quality of life benefits for the patient). Recommend that families discuss options with surgeons (including those performing periodontal surgery) and anesthesiologists/anesthetists. Such options might include avoiding cerebral effects of general anesthesia or conscious sedation by use of local or regional anesthesia for cooperative patients or else at least minimizing dosages of medications used for general anesthesia and conscious sedation. That said, patients with advanced dementia who are unable to cooperate with necessary procedures or might harm themselves or the medical professionals during such operations (e.g. to address an abscessed tooth) may require something in the way of general anesthesia or conscious sedation.

Stages of dementia

A variety of classification schemes denote stages of dementia. Perhaps the easiest and most straightforward framework is one categorizing mild, moderate, severe, and late stages. These have been most widely studied in AD, but can be extrapolated to other types of dementia. In the case of AD, patients with mild-stage illness might have memory difficulties that interfere with their performance of instrumental activities of daily living (IADLs), such as managing finances or grocery shopping, and may have minor impairment of other cognitive domains, but maintain appropriate social behavior and can carry out basic ADLs (BADLs). Most patients with dementia come to the attention of a specialist, such as a neurologist, in the moderate stage of disease. Patients with moderate-stage AD may have significant deficits in memory and other cognitive impairments impeding daily function as well as noticeable behavioral problems, such as agitation.

Herein, reference to advanced dementia signifies severe or late-stage dementia. Severe dementia indicates global cognitive impairment and dependency upon others for most ADLs. Given age and other medical factors, many patients with dementia do not survive to late-stage dementia. That is to say,

many patients with dementia are elderly and die, like most Americans, of stroke or heart attack. Those patients that do enter late-stage dementia are typically dependent on others for all ADLs, totally incontinent (of bowel and bladder), severely cognitively impaired (e.g. may not be able to state their full name or recognize close family members), and require 24-h supervision and often skilled nursing care. Neurologists are unlikely to see patients with late-stage dementia in an office setting, but may do so as hospital consultants or if they call on patients in long-term care facilities.

Be sure not to confuse mild-stage dementia with early-onset dementia. A patient who has the onset of dementia before 65 years of age has early-onset dementia, but will go through all the stages of dementia if they live long enough. Therefore, the term mild stage is preferred over early stage to indicate the beginning phase of dementia, while early onset is reserved for those patients who have dementia starting at a younger age. (Perhaps "young onset" would be an even clearer way to state this.)

Recent clinical consensus guidelines for dementia include mild cognitive impairment (MCI) under the rubric of preclinical AD. Patients with MCI convert to AD at a rate of 12–15% per annum and 80% have converted to AD after 5 years. Thus, it is wise to prepare such patients and families for this high chance of conversion and give them a chance for advance planning, to consider options for medical intervention, and opportunities for research participation.

Prognosis

Almost every family brings up this question, which suggests that those that don't probably are just afraid to ask. Therefore, it should be addressed, but consider that some may not want to know (or be ready for) the answer. For the most part, let a family's questions guide the discussion. And of course, answer those from patients, although many don't have questions, perhaps due to apathy or difficulties in complex abstract reasoning.

So, what do you tell them? After defining dementia and giving the patient a specific dementia diagnosis based on history, examination, and neuroimaging or other testing, it may help to start with a positive spin: dementia generally worsens slowly over years, not days or weeks or even months. (This generally holds true except for the rare rapidly progressive dementias, such as Creutzfeldt–Jakob and other prion diseases.) Point out the importance of diagnosis in providing an explanation for changes in a patient's thinking, behavior, and function and make it clear that a patient has a specific brain disease. Advise that other factors, including other medical conditions, will play a part in the patient's course and longevity.

Many families press for a specific answer, often with extremely valid reasons, such as limited funds for care, etc. The earlier in the course of dementia, the less accurate the prediction, and it depends on dementia subtype as well as many other individual factors. Taking that into account, the median time of survival from onset of disease symptoms is ~10 years in AD and ~7 years in FTD. Vascular and mixed (Alzheimer's+vascular) dementia tend to be much more variable due to the nature of these diseases and associated cardiac and other medical conditions.

Work with families to help avoid procedures which may be non-essential, futile, or even harmful for patients in advanced stages of dementia (this includes screening evaluations, such as colonoscopies, mammograms, and dental, gynecological, and prostate exams). As patients enter later stages of dementia, inform families of symptoms, such as severe weight loss, total incontinence, mutism, and severe loss of mobility, which may indicate an evaluation for hospice care in advanced dementia. (See Chapter 9 regarding palliative care in advanced dementia.)

Follow-up assessment

The ABCD of dementia

Categorizing dementia symptoms provides a useful framework within which to evaluate stage of dementia, progression, and goals of therapy. Information should be obtained from family caregivers (perhaps in writing, as described above, especially for embarrassing or possibly volatile topics) regarding a patient's functioning, mood and behavior, and cognition. In each of these categories, ask about trends of decline, stabilization, or (less likely) improvement since a prior visit. Caregiver perception of rates of decline may also be helpful if these can be ascertained (e.g. is a patient's function/behavior/memory declining more, less, or the same since medication was started?). Some physicians may find it useful to utilize a questionnaire, such as

the AD8 (see Chapter 6), which can be completed by a family caregiver in the waiting room.

Activities of daily living (ADLs)

As described previously, IADLs comprise complex tasks, such as driving and meal preparation whereas BADLs include daily self-care such as dressing and hygiene.

Behavior and mood

Behavioral problems in dementia may include agitation, aggression, and aberrant motor behavior (pacing, wandering, etc.). Mood issues include anxiety, irritability, apathy, and depression. Psychosis includes hallucinations and/or delusions, which may also be accompanied by agitation.

Cognition

Although neurologists and other physicians often focus on the cognitive assessment of patients with dementia, this is often the least of a caregiver's worries. It is not essential to perform comprehensive neuropsychological assessment for clinical follow-up of a patient. In fact, it is often better to avoid this, unless needed as part of research, to minimize stressing a patient. One quick test is the Mini-Cog in which a patient repeats three words, performs the clock drawing task, and then must recall the three words given. It has been validated as a dementia screening test. It can be used as a follow-up test and, for example, clock drawings may be compared, but it is so short as to be limited as a follow-up tool. Neurologists may find it useful to perform mental status testing, such as the Montreal Cognitive Assessment (MOCA), which is available in the public domain and includes tasks of executive functioning or the Folstein Mini-Mental State Examination (MMSE) ©, along with a test of executive functioning, such as the clock drawing task (since the Folstein MMSE provides little information regarding this cognitive domain). Physicians may also create their own formal or informal short list of questions and/or tasks. Neurologists must be sure to ask the exact date and year rather than assume it is remembered or forgotten. Asking a patient to recall their birthdate and age are also quite telling questions and the answers may direct recommendations regarding a patient's need for assistance with ADLs and decision making.

What is most important is to assess a few cognitive domains, especially memory, visuospatial skills, and executive functioning (particularly for any patients who may be driving). Some language may be assessed in conversation, but this necessitates letting the patient speak for themselves (rather than the caregiver).

Delay nursing home placement

Antidementia medications may help in this regard, but easing caregiver burden represents an important bulwark of this goal. Ask caregivers how they are doing and offer support, resources, and care options, including referring them back to their physicians or to a therapist, support group, or community organization, if you cannot fully address their needs. Caregivers of patients with dementia are more likely to experience depression than caregivers of patients with other illnesses and should receive professional assessment and treatment for suspected depression.

☆ TIPS AND TRICKS

Follow up on mood, behavioral, and functional issues with family caregivers as these problems frequently result in increased caregiver burden, hospitalization, or other institutionalization, and may often be addressed by a multimodal approach, including non-pharmacological measures, or with medication, when other intervention fails.

Planning

As the foregoing sections make clear, a little preparation goes a long way. Counseling patients and families regarding planning is one of the most important aspects of dementia care. Early diagnosis facilitates such care and planning.

Patients and families should seek to put legal and monetary affairs in order, preferably with professional advice (e.g. from attorneys, financial planners, etc.). Wills, powers of attorney (POA), and advance healthcare directives (including MPOA and living wills) should be executed while a person has the capacity to do so. The costly legal process of guardianship is not necessary for most patients and may often be avoided by such advance planning. While not legally required, a frank discussion of end-of-life care

between patients and family (or other medical decision makers) may help ease anxieties and make sure a patient's wishes are honored.

Such planning and preparation may be important not just for patients, but for close loved ones. Those who have already ordered their legal affairs are to be commended, but these may need to be revisited, particularly in the case of spousal caregivers or others who may have a loved one with dementia listed as a durable POA or MPOA or executor of a will. Even patients with dementia who might currently serve in such a role might be unable to fulfill it in the future. Patients diagnosed with dementia or MCI will be unlikely to obtain long-term care insurance coverage, but it may be possible (and wise) for their primary family caregiver (such as a spouse) to do so.

Driving and other safety issues

Driving

If the patient is still driving, a responsible adult family member should monitor their driving every couple of weeks or so. This means riding as a passenger in the car to the places which the patient usually drives to, without giving directions, and assessing driving safety. Studies show that if the family doesn't think a loved one with dementia can drive safely, the patient probably can't, whereas if a patient thinks himself or herself safe to drive, this self-assessment is unreliable. Each case is individual. Some states require reporting of patients with dementia (including MCI). You should check and know the requirements, if any, for the area in which you practice. Such reporting requirements actually help ease the burden of doctors and caregivers by shifting the onus for assessment, etc. to the state. Even the suggestion of revoking driving privileges based on cognitive impairment is often more difficult for patients than receiving a diagnosis of dementia! Some patients may have other reasons, such as poor vision, weakness, back or leg pain, loss of insurance coverage due to dementia diagnosis, etc. which they may find a more palatable explanation than cognitive impairment as to why they may no longer drive. Some patients may drive safely but require another family member to navigate. These patients should not be allowed to drive alone. However, this restriction may convey a mixed and confusing message to a patient with cognitive impairment. It may be safer and easier for a family to arrange for a patient not to drive at all, rather than with some restrictions.

Recommend that the household in which the patient lives has a number of cars commensurate with the number of drivers and to avoid leaving a vehicle, particularly one a patient used to drive, clearly visible (i.e. best to park the car in the garage rather than in plain sight on the driveway).

Weapons and hunting

Patients with dementia may need limited access to firearms or other weapons or proximity to others with such weapons (especially patients who have difficulty following instructions and might have problems staying out of harm's way in an environment where others are shooting or hunting). Appropriate precautions should be taken when patients or others may be at potential risk of harm. This includes locking, unloading, or even removal of such weapons as well as discontinuing any hunting or gun licenses.

Other safety issues

A variety of safety issues may arise. A common theme is a need for increased supervision to prevent harm, which must be addressed. For example, a patient who continually forgets to take medications (or otherwise takes them incorrectly) may be at increased risk of an inadequately treated medical condition and/or adverse effects due to erratic dosing. Increased assistance with medication administration should be provided. A patient who doesn't know what to do in case of a fire (e.g. can't recall to dial 911 in an emergency) should not be left alone. This scenario may easily be posed as a hypothetical question to a patient in the medical setting.

Neuroimaging, laboratory testing, and other tests

Neuroimaging, laboratory testing, and comprehensive neuropsychological testing may be useful in initial diagnosis. However, these need not be repeated unless a patient exhibits a sudden change in mental status or other neurological sign or symptom that indicates need for assessment independent of dementia. Patients with dementia may have delirium superimposed on dementia, strokes, or infection, and are at a higher risk of seizures than age-matched controls. Unless a patient

with dementia is designated as comfort care only or enrolled in palliative or hospice care, mental status changes and other neurological symptoms should be assessed just as they would be for any other patient (e.g. a delirium work-up including a urinalysis to check for urinary tract infection as a potential etiology of new-onset psychosis in an elderly individual). Avoid tests that will not change management and avoid procedures that will not improve quality of life, particularly in patients with advanced dementia (see Chapter 9 for further discussion). Age and dementia confer higher risk of seizures and work-up (including electroencephalogram) and/or intervention may be indicated.

Hospitalization

This can be overwhelming for anyone, but particularly the patient with dementia. Having family members organize a schedule allowing each to take shifts staying with the patient can facilitate communication (including reminding staff to "start low and go slow" with new medications) and allow use of non-pharmacological measures (such as talking and reassurance from a familiar person) for behavioral decompensation.

Genetics and prevention

Genetic testing is not indicated for asymptomatic patients. It is also unnecessary for the clinical care of most patients with dementia. Genetic testing may be considered for patients with dementia with an onset age less than age 65 and/or a strong family history of dementia. Such cases might be referred to a subspecialist, such as a behavioral or geriatric neurologist or geriatric psychiatrist, or to a dementia research center. The assistance of a genetic counselor is invaluable.

Family members often inquire about their chances of developing dementia and, for those who don't, this may be an unspoken concern. For most patients with dementia (barring the exceptions noted in the previous paragraph), age is the biggest risk factor for dementia. Therefore, most patients with dementia are healthy enough to live into their 70s and 80s. That is to say, those individuals who are long-lived have a greater risk for dementia. Therefore, family members may only get dementia if they live to a ripe old age. They actually have "good" genes in terms of longevity.

Comparison to another familiar disease condition may be useful. For example, heart attacks may "run" in some families, but rarely is a single gene linked to this problem. Rather, it is a complex interplay of genetics and environment. To take the example of AD in monozygotic ("identical") twins, if one has AD, the other has only a one in three chance of having this disease.

A corollary concern to genetics (and one that is also commonly raised or at the top of a family member's mind) is the issue of prevention. Regardless of the type of dementia, this author usually tells families (and others) that the top three things that they can do to help prevent it are: *control vascular risk factors, control vascular risk factors, control vascular risk factors*. This is followed by specifically outlining what these factors are (e.g. smoking, hypertension, cholesterol, diabetes, obesity). If patients have vitamin deficiencies or similar abnormalities (e.g. vitamin B12 or D deficiency or hyperhomocysteinemia), recommend that their blood relatives are also checked for these treatable conditions which can variously pose risks for dementia, other neurological illness, and/or vascular disease.

Those patients and families who have a family history of dementia or are very interested in genetics and/or prevention are excellent candidates for participation in research. This option should be discussed and a referral made for those who are interested.

Refer for research

Our understanding of dementia has expanded greatly, in no small part due to the contributions of thousands of participants in clinical research. However, we have much more to learn and medications for dementia leave much to be desired. Most dementia research is done in AD, but opportunities exist for family members, people with normal memory, and patients with other types of dementia.

Therefore, encourage and refer patients, caregivers, families, and others for research. Such a referral might be to the National Institutes of Health (NIH) website (www.clinicaltrials.gov), the Alzheimer's Association clinical trials program (known as TrialMatch™, under the Clinical Trials tab at www.alz.org/research), or local research centers (including the nationwide Alzheimer's Disease Centers which conduct research into a variety of dementias and can be located via www.nia.nih.gov/Alzheimers).

Helping the helper

This includes not just the primary family caregiver, but a patient's physicians as well. Familiarize yourself with websites or phone numbers of local resources. Many organizations will be happy to supply your office with materials, so that you may provide patients and caregivers with the information they need in a waiting room or patient library. You should also keep a supply close at hand, so that you can choose the most relevant brochure, say one addressing problem behaviors or respite care, for specific situations.

Care options

Caregiving works best as a team approach and if a primary family caregiver is not the *sole* caregiver. The involvement of professional and other caregivers, including family and friends, may prevent or postpone institutionalization. However, when this can no longer be deferred, the choice is not necessarily a stark one between home or nursing home, despite common misconceptions.

It behooves physicians to inform families of the gamut of care options that may help keep a patient living at home as well as the plethora of residential care choices that now exist. Social workers, geriatric care managers , and community organizations are typically quite knowledgeable about local resources. Assistance from a social worker may be covered as part of hospitalization or home health.

Speaking of home health, such services, as covered by Medicare and other health insurance, are usually too limited to offer substantial caregiver relief and should not be a substitute for the more long-term and expanded help discussed below (which Medicare and other health insurance do not cover, although long-term care insurance might).

Professional caregiver support includes adult day programs, which patients and families are often more receptive to if they are introduced as "brain therapy." These are conducted by long-term care facilities and community-based centers and allow a patient to get out of the home, socialize, and participate in group activities, while giving the caregiver a break. Respite care may be provided by private agencies at home or offered by long-term care facilities. This allows patients temporary 24-h care and affords caregivers a chance to do such things as go out of town when a patient can no longer travel or just get a break for a few days to weeks. It may be covered by veterans' benefits in some cases. The cost of full-time in-home care may be prohibitive for many, but a few hours care on an intermittent but regular basis may mean the difference between a patient living at home or requiring permanent placement.

Long-term care placement options include assisted living, memory care (also called Alzheimer's care or assisted living-plus), and skilled nursing care facilities. It makes no sense for a patient with dementia who can no longer live independently at home to move to independent living. Sometimes assisted living also may not be enough. Families should carefully explore options via websites, other resources (such as printed materials) available locally, and community organizations and visit any potential facility (preferably several times) and talk with other residents and families there. If a patient with dementia has a spouse or other family member also moving to such a facility, it may be helpful to choose one with different levels of care to accommodate the needs of both.

Conclusion

Neurologists can play an important role in the care of patients with dementia, as well as their families, ensuring that none has to travel this path alone or unguided.

Further reading

Albert M, DeKosky ST, Dickson D, et al. The diagnosis of mild cognitive impairment due to Alzheimer's disease: report of the National Institute on Aging and the Alzheimer's Association workgroup. *Alzheimers Dement* 2011; **7**(3): 270–9.

Borson S, Scanlan JM, Chen P, Ganguli M. The Mini-Cog as a screen for dementia: validation in a population-based sample. *J Am Geriatr Soc* 2003; **51**(10): 1451–4.

Galvin JE, Roe CM, Powlishta KK, et al. The AD8: a brief informant interview to detect dementia. *Neurology* 2005; **65**(4): 559–64.

Goldman JS, Hahn SE, Catania JW, et al. Genetic counseling and testing for Alzheimer disease: joint practice guidelines of the American College of Medical Genetics and the National Society of Genetic Counselors. *Genet Med* 2011; **13**(6): 597–605.

Iverson DJ, Gronseth GS, Reger MA, et al., for the Quality Standards Subcomitee of the American Academy of Neurology. Practice parameter update: evaluation and management of driving risk in dementia: report of the Quality Standards Subcommittee of the American Academy of Neurology. *Neurology* 2010; **74**(16): 1316–24.

Knopman DS, DeKosky ST, Cummings JL, et al. Practice parameter: diagnosis of dementia (an evidence-based review). Report of the Quality Standards Subcommittee of the American Academy of Neurology. *Neurology* 2001; **56**(9): 1143–53.

Lipton AM, Marshall CD. *The Common Sense Guide to Dementia for Clinicians and Caregivers*. New York: Springer, 2012.

McKhann GM, Knopman DS, Chertkow H, et al. The diagnosis of dementia due to Alzheimer's disease: recommendations from the National Institute on Aging and the Alzheimer's Association workgroup. *Alzheimers Dement* 2011; **7**(3): 263–9.

Petersen RC. Conversion. *Neurology* 2006; **67**: S12–13.

Sperling RA, Aisen PS, Beckett LA, et al. Toward defining the preclinical stages of Alzheimer's disease: recommendations from the National Institute on Aging-Alzheimer's Association workgroups on diagnostic guidelines for Alzheimer's disease. *Alzheimers Dement* 2011; **7**(3): 280–92.

Tariot PN, Farlow MR, Grossberg GT, et al., for the Memantine Study Group. Memantine treatment in patients with moderate to severe Alzheimer disease already receiving donepezil: a randomized controlled trial. *JAMA* 2004; **291**(3): 317–24.

Weiner MF, Lipton AM (eds). *The Dementias: Diagnosis, Treatment and Research*, 3rd edn. Washington, DC: American Psychiatric Publishing, 2003.

Weiner MF, Lipton AM (eds). *The American Psychiatric Publishing Textbook of Alzheimer Disease and Other Dementias*. Washington, DC: American Psychiatric Publishing, 2009.

Weiner MF, Lipton AM (eds). *Clinical Manual of Alzheimer Disease and Other Dementias*. Washington, DC: American Psychiatric Publishing, 2012.

Websites

Alzheimer's Assocation: www.alz.org

Association for Frontotemporal Degeneration: www.theaftd.org

Caring.com: www.caring.com

Lewy Body Dementia Association: www.lbda.org

National Institutes of Health/Alzheimer's Disease Centers: www.nia.nih.gov/Alzheimers

National Institutes of Health: www.nih.gov (A–Z listing of diseases is particularly helpful), www.clinical trials.gov

8

Using Psychotropic Medications to Manage Problem Behaviors in Dementia

Lucy Y. Wang and Murray A. Raskind

Department of Psychiatry and Behavioral Sciences, University of Washington, USA

Introduction

Although dementia is primarily considered a cognitive disorder, non-cognitive or behavioral symptoms also develop in almost all patients at some point during their illness. Depression and apathy often emerge in early-stage dementia. Hallucinations, delusions, agitation, and sleep disturbance commonly occur in later stage illness. These symptoms, and particularly agitation, are difficult to manage at home and in the long-term care facility alike. Patients are in distress, caregivers experience burnout, and behaviors often precipitate admission to long-term care facilities. Successful treatment can improve the quality of lives for patients and caregivers.

However, finding the best treatment strategy can be challenging. Psychotropic medications may be only partly effective and have side-effects that limit the dose or length of treatment. Often the choice of psychotropic medication is empirical, based on individual symptoms and treatment response. The best treatment approach usually involves an individualized combination of non-pharmacological and pharmacological methods.

This chapter provides information that can aid clinicians in developing these treatment strategies to help their patients. Chapter content will highlight the more common behavioral symptoms seen in dementia: agitation and aggression, psychosis, sleep disturbance, depression, and apathy. The bulk of the discussion will relate to treatments useful in Alzheimer's disease (AD), but most medication strategies can be applied to other dementia types. Exceptions will be specifically described, including symptoms or medications unique to Parkinson's disease dementia (PDD), dementia with Lewy bodies (DLB), vascular dementia, and behavioral-variant frontotemporal dementia (bvFTD).

General treatment approach

Before considering a medication to treat a problem behavior in dementia, always attempt a non-pharmacological treatment either before or in combination with medications. There are many non-pharmacological approaches available and descriptions of all of these exceed the scope of the chapter. However, some approaches easily implemented during an office visit are summarized in Box 8.1.

> **⚠ CAUTION**
>
> When assessing a problem behavior for the first time, also look into causes other than dementia. For example, untreated pain, a medication side-effect or delirium can cause agitation, depression or hallucinations.

When non-pharmacological approaches have been tried and yet symptoms persist, medication trials are then recommended. The choice of medication depends on the specific symptom targets,

Dementia, First Edition. Edited by Joseph F. Quinn.

the severity of symptoms, and side-effect profiles. Because efficacy is usually only modest, it is important to discuss with families realistic expectations for improvement and continue using non-pharmacological measures. Also keep in mind that the natural course of many symptoms is to resolve later during the dementia illness, so careful reductions in doses or even discontinuation of medications can be attempted after a period of stability.

★ **TIPS AND TRICKS**

A common mantra for dosing medications in geriatric populations is "start low and go slow." Geriatric psychiatry is no exception. A reasonable rule of thumb is to start a psychiatric medication at half the usual adult dose and increase slowly over weeks rather than days, until the lowest effective dose is reached. However, some patients may require doses in the higher range to manage symptoms adequately.

Box 8.1 Some non-pharmacological approaches to problem behaviors in dementia

Provide caregiver support.
  Education about the disease, course, and prognosis.
  Referral to a support group network or advocacy group (e.g. Alzheimer's Association).
  Assess need for additional help (e.g. other family members, paid caregivers, adult day health, respite programs).

Suggest changes to a patient's environment.

  Reduce overstimulation (e.g. turn off television, move bedroom to a quieter area).
  Set up a calmer atmosphere (e.g. relaxing music, aromatherapy).
  Improve daytime lighting.
  Add healthy activities.
  Exercise.
  Art or recreation therapy.
  Social visits from family or volunteers.
  Structured activities (e.g. senior center, adult day health).

Agitation and aggression

Agitation and aggression are terms used to describe a cluster of symptoms where patients are physically or verbally overactive in a way that is distressing to themselves or those around them. Symptoms can be in mild forms such as pressured pacing, difficulty sitting still, and irritability. They can also be severe, where examples include throwing objects and physically assaulting others. Agitation and aggression result in compromised access to care, hospitalizations, or admissions to long-term care settings. Therefore appropriate treatments are imperative for the quality of life and safety of both patients and caregivers. Pharmacological treatment options for agitation are summarized in Table 8.1, and include the cholinesterase inhibitors, memantine, antidepressants, atypical antipsychotics, adrenergic antagonists, and benzodiazepines. Specifics are discussed below.

Mild agitation

Cholinesterase inhibitors and memantine

Non-pharmacological approaches are recommended for mild agitation, because mild agitation is more likely to respond to non-medication strategies, and because the side-effects of most drugs used to treat agitation outweigh the potential benefit. However, the primary agents used for cognition, cholinesterase inhibitors and memantine, may be of

Table 8.1 Medication choices for dementia-related agitation

Agitation characteristics	Medication choices	Time to response
Infrequent Minimal distress Redirectable	Cholinesterase inhibitors Memantine Selective serotonin reuptake inhibitors	Weeks
Frequent Significant distress Interferes with necessary care	Atypical antipsychotics Prazosin	Days to weeks
Physical aggression (hitting, kicking, throwing things) The safety of the patient or others is at risk	Atypical antipsychotics Benzodiazepines Anticonvulsants	Days

some utility. Post hoc analyses have shown that Alzheimer's disease patients taking cholinesterase inhibitors (donepezil, rivastigmine, and galantamine) and memantine have had less severe or fewer behavioral symptoms than patients taking placebo. However, it is important to realize that persons with moderate or severe behavior symptoms were excluded from these studies. The cholinesterase inhibitors are also indicated for vascular dementia, DLB, and PDD. As these medications already are recommended for their cognitive effects, it is worthwhile establishing adequate trials of these drugs if patients are also exhibiting mild agitation.

Contraindications to cholinesterase inhibitors include severe liver or lung disease, bradycardia, and severe peptic ulcer disease. Prominent side-effects are nausea and diarrhea, which can be minimized by very slow upward titrations no more quickly than every 4–6 weeks. Memantine is an N-methyl-D-aspartate (NMDA) receptor antagonist and is indicated for moderate-to-severe Alzheimer's disease. This medication is generally well tolerated with few side-effects. In some individuals, there may be a transient worsening in confusion.

Antidepressants

Antidepressant medications that have been studied for dementia-related agitation include the selective serotonin reuptake inhibitors (SSRI) and trazodone (Tables 8.2 and 8.3). Results are mixed, and there-

Table 8.2 Selective serotonin reuptake inhibitors

Medication	How supplied	Dosing	Remarks
Citalopram	Oral solution, tablet	5–20 mg daily	Has few drug–drug interactions; common side-effects are nausea and somnolence; a rare but serious side-effect is dose-related prolongation of the QT interval
Sertraline	Oral solution, tablet	25–200 mg daily	Has few drug–drug interactions; common side-effects are diarrhea, nausea, and insomnia
Fluoxetine	Capsule, oral solution, syrup, tablet	5–40 mg daily	Multiple medication interactions; long half-life (4–6 days); common side-effects are nausea and insomnia
Paroxetine	Tablet, oral suspension	5–40 mg daily	Multiple medication interactions; common side-effects are nausea, insomnia, and somnolence

Table 8.3 Other antidepressants

Medication	Mechanism of action	Dose	Remarks
Mirtazapine	Enhances noradrenergic and serotonergic activity	7.5–60 mg at bedtime	Due to sedating properties, may be helpful for concomitant sleep disturbance
Venlafaxine	Serotonin norepinephrine reuptake inhibitor	37.5–150 mg daily in divided doses (once daily with the extended-release formulation)	Higher doses are associated with elevations in blood pressure
Duloxetine	Serotonin norepinephrine reuptake inhibitor	30–60 mg once daily	Also FDA indicated for chronic musculoskeletal pain, fibromyalgia, and neuropathic pain
Trazodone	Serotonin antagonist and reuptake inhibitor	25–250 mg at bedtime	Sedating, often also used as a sleep aid; can cause priapism

fore they are a potential option for treatment in individualized cases but not routinely recommended by treatment guidelines. They may be considered for patients with milder symptoms or those who do not tolerate or do not respond to antipsychotics.

Moderate to severe agitation and aggression

Antipsychotics

For more severe degrees of agitation, in which distress or risk to the patient and caregivers requires immediate intervention, antipsychotics are the agents with demonstrated, albeit modest, efficacy. Because of a high adverse effect burden of the older ("typical," e.g. haloperidol) antipsychotics, the second-generation ("atypical") antipsychotics are preferred. The atypical antipsychotic medications that have been studied for dementia-related agitation include olanzapine, risperidone, quetiapine, and aripiprazole.

Unfortunately, the side-effects of the atypical antipsychotics are also significant and limit their use. These include sedation, falls, and extrapyramidal symptoms. These drugs can cause metabolic syndrome, but this problem is of less concern in the elderly dementia population than younger persons. Older adults are also particularly vulnerable to extrapyramidal symptoms, such as parkinsonism and tardive dyskinesia.

EVIDENCE AT A GLANCE

Placebo-controlled trials of the typical antipsychotics risperidone, olanzapine, quetiapine, and aripiprazole demonstrated modest efficacy for agitation and aggression in AD, and were moderately well tolerated at low doses. However, a major study comparing several atypical antipsychotics head to head, the CATIE-AD study, demonstrated less promising results. In this study, patients with dementia-related agitation or psychosis were given placebo, olanzapine, risperidone, or quetiapine. Researchers discovered that although olanzapine and risperidone reduced some symptoms, their side-effects still caused patients and their doctors to want to stop the medication. Their conclusion was that the medications' overall effectiveness, when side-effects were taken into account, was not different from placebo.

A notable concern is an increased risk of death associated with antipsychotic drug use in dementia patients with agitation and psychosis, which is the basis for a Food and Drug Administration (FDA) black box warning against use of these agents. A 2005 analyses of 17 atypical antipsychotic placebo-controlled trials that enrolled 5377 elderly patients with dementia-related behavioral disorders found an approximately 1.6–1.7-fold increase in mortality rate (4.5%, compared with 2.6% in the patients taking placebo). In 2008 the FDA expanded the black box warning to first-generation antipsychotics as well, based on two large retrospective studies indicating that risk of mortality associated with first-generation antipsychotics was comparable to or exceeded that of the atypicals. Some data suggest that sedation is associated with this increased mortality.

Although there is a negative side-effect profile and increased risk associated with atypical antipsychotics, there is also significant risk to inadequate treatment of agitation. In many situations where a patient's agitation and aggression are endangering themselves or others, the benefits of use often outweigh risks. Many patients and families also express a willingness to accept a small increased risk if the patient's quality of life meaningfully improves with antipsychotic treatment. For these reasons atypical antipsychotics are still commonly used and included in treatment guidelines. Information specific to each atypical antipsychotic is summarized in Table 8.4.

✋ CAUTION

Because antipsychotics increase the risk of mortality in dementia patients (which is described in an FDA black box warning), it is imperative that the risks and benefits of treatment be carefully discussed with patients and families.

The question of how long to continue antipsychotic medications remains unclear. While agitation will persist in many patients, it may resolve spontaneously and not recur in others. Therefore it is important to carefully evaluate the ongoing need for these drugs, including attempts at dose reduction. For nursing homes, the Centers for Medicare and Medicaid Services have published guidelines that delineate a timeline for gradual dose reduction,

Table 8.4 Atypical antipsychotics that have demonstrated modest efficacy for dementia-related agitation and aggression in most studies

Medication	How supplied	Starting dose (mg)	Dosing frequency	Dose range (mg/day)
Risperidone	Tablet, oral solution, disintegrating tablet	0.25	Once to twice daily	0.25–2
Olanzapine	Tablet, disintegrating tablet	2.5	Once daily	2.5–10
Quetiapine	Tablet, extended-release tablet	12.5	Once to three times daily	12.5–200
Aripiprazole	Tablet, oral solution, disintegrating tablet	2.5	Once daily	2.5–15

where within the first year an antipsychotic medication is initiated, there must be at least two attempts at gradual dose reduction with at least 1 month between attempts. After the first year, gradual dose reduction should be attempted on an annual basis.

Adrenergic receptor antagonists

The pathophysiology underlying agitation and aggression remains to be fully elucidated, but emerging evidence in AD research suggests that an abnormal compensatory upregulation in noradrenergic activity may be a contributing factor. This substantiates the rationale that medications which dampen noradrenergic responsiveness, such as adrenergic receptor antagonists (Table 8.5), are of benefit.

Specifically, increased numbers of alpha-1 adrenoreceptors in rostral locus ceruleus projection areas have been associated with antemortem agitation and aggression in AD. This finding provides a rationale for alpha-1 adrenoreceptor antagonists in the treatment of agitation in AD. It is worth noting that all the antipsychotics discussed above have substantial alpha-1 adrenoreceptor antagonist activity. The alpha-1 adrenoreceptor antagonist prazosin provides a more potent and less complex approach to reducing brain alpha-1 adrenoreceptor responsiveness in the agitated AD patient. Recently, a double-blind placebo-controlled pilot study demonstrated that prazosin effectively improved behavioral symptoms in agitated AD patients with minimal blood pressure reduction or adverse effects. Although this study was small, clinical trials are ongoing. Prazosin's relatively benign, non-sedating side-effect profile, especially when compared to the atypical antipsychotics, makes it an attractive treatment alternative. Side-effects to monitor include lower extremity edema and orthostatic hypotension.

Table 8.5 Adrenergic antagonists

Medication	Dose	Remarks
Prazosin	Start with 1 mg daily, and increase as needed by 1–2 mg every 3–7 days, up to 10 mg twice daily	Monitor for orthostatic hypotension
Propranolol	10 mg 3 times a day, and gradually increase as needed up to 40 mg 3 times a day	May lower blood pressure and pulse; contraindications include hypotension, bradycardia, bronchospastic pulmonary disease, and diabetes mellitus

The beta-blocker propranolol has also been used for treating agitation and aggression in dementia. However, a study of propranolol, although showing modest efficacy, also revealed that it is limited by hypotension and bradycardia. Propranolol's efficacy may decline over time as well.

> ★ **TIPS AND TRICKS**
>
> The likelihood of prazosin causing hypotension decreases when it is started at 1 mg per day and increased slowly, based on clinical response. If a blood pressure decrease causes concern after a prazosin dose increase, one can reduce the dose and attempt an increase at a later date.

Anticonvulsants

Carbamazepine and valproic acid have been studied as treatments for dementia-related agitation. Results are mixed and side-effects, particularly sedation and gait disturbance, can be problematic. Therefore anticonvulsants are not routinely recommended. However, trials of either of these agents may be considered, particularly in situations where a patient is physically aggressive and does not tolerate or respond to antipsychotic agents. When prescribing carbamazepine or valproic acid, titrate to clinical response and not to blood level. Patients usually respond to doses lower than those used for seizure disorders.

Benzodiazepines

Benzodiazepines are frequently prescribed for dementia-related agitation, although side-effects also limit their usefulness. These side-effects include sedation, increased risk of falls, delirium, and disinhibition that paradoxically worsens agitation. Therefore long-term use is best avoided, although short-term or rare occasional use may be appropriate (e.g. agitation related to a dental procedure or a diagnostic study, agitation so severe that there is risk of harm to self or others). Also, agents with shorter half-lives and fewer or no metabolites are preferred, such as lorazepam or oxazepam (Table 8.6).

★ TIPS AND TRICKS

Benzodiazepines are known to sometimes cause "paradoxical" reactions, when instead of reducing agitation they can worsen it. It is important to monitor response carefully when starting a benzodiazepine. Also, when evaluating someone with agitation currently prescribed a benzodiazepine, a good first step is trying a gradual dose reduction.

Hallucinations and delusions

Hallucinations and delusions, which are referred to collectively as psychosis, are also common occurrences in dementia. In AD, these symptoms usually emerge late in the disease. Hallucinations may be auditory or visual. Delusions tend to be simple, non-bizarre and of a paranoid nature. Examples include the belief that caregivers are stealing from them, misidentification of caregivers, or a belief that their

Table 8.6 Benzodiazepines with shorter half-lives or fewer metabolites, preferred in older adults

Medication	How supplied	Dosing
Lorazepam	Oral solution, tablet	0.5–1 mg every 4–6 h on an as-needed basis, standing doses of 0.5–1 mg may be given 1–4 times per day
Oxazepam	Capsule	Standing doses of 7.5–15 mg may be given 1–4 times per day

current living situation is not really their home. It can often be difficult to determine whether delusions represent a true psychotic process or a patient's misinterpretation of their surroundings due to their memory impairment.

In DLB, visual hallucinations are a diagnostic criterion and can occur much earlier in the disease course. Visual hallucinations are also common in PDD. In both of these syndromes, visual hallucinations usually start as benign images, such as of small children or animals. Patients maintain insight that their visions are not reality based, and therefore are typically not distressed by them. However, as their dementia progresses, their hallucinations can become threatening and they can lose insight. Delusions similar to those experienced by AD patients can also occur in DLB and PDD.

If the hallucinations or delusions are not distressing to the patient, it is better not to treat with medications. These symptoms are often more distressing to loved ones and caregivers than patients themselves, so careful education about the nature of these symptoms and finding non-pharmacological adaptation strategies provide more benefit. For PDD patients, decreasing or changing dopaminergic medications is a good first step because these drugs can produce psychotic symptoms. It is also important to determine whether a delusion may in fact represent cognitive impairment rather than a true psychotic symptom. If cognitive, a cholinesterase inhibitor or memantine may be helpful.

If psychotic symptoms are distressing to patients and impair their quality of life, an atypical antipsychotic can be useful. However, antipsychotic treatment is tempered by limited efficacy, side-effects, and the increased risk of mortality associated with these drugs as described in the section above on agitation. For AD patients, the medications and dosage ranges described in Table 8.4 are recommended. For DLB and PDD patients, antipsychotic use is complicated by the high potential to worsen their already present parkinsonian symptoms. The two medications least likely to worsen parkinsonism are clozapine and quetiapine. Clozapine carries a risk for agranulocytosis, and therefore requires prescribers to have specific training and access to appropriate monitoring with weekly blood tests. Quetiapine is therefore more commonly used. Finally, it is important to discuss and document the potential risks versus benefits of any antipsychotic with patients and caregivers, including the FDA black box warning for increased mortality risk.

Sleep disturbance

Sleep disturbance is common in dementia and is one of the primary reasons patients move from home to long-term care facilities. Sleep pattern changes vary, involving a range of nighttime awakenings, decreased overall sleep time, increased daytime napping, or shifts in the sleep/wake cycle.

Non pharmacological approaches are again recommended as first line for sleep disturbance. Education for caregivers about implementing sleep hygiene can be helpful, including establishing regular sleep and wake times, increasing daytime activities, and starting calming nighttime rituals. If patients are in a facility with adequate staffing at night, simply allowing the patient to be awake at night is also a reasonable approach. Another important step is reviewing patients' medical conditions. Sleep apnea is common in dementia patients and is a relative contraindication for sedative-hypnotics that decrease respiratory drive. Medication side-effects can also impair sleep. Diphenhydramine, often used to aid sleep, may in fact worsen sleep in dementia patients because of anticholinergic effects.

If choosing a medication primarily utilized for sleep disturbance, non-benzodiazepines are preferred because benzodiazepines increase the risk of falls, disinhibition, and delirium. Many clinicians prefer trazodone. Other non-benzodiazepine options include zolpidem, zaleplon, and eszopiclone.

Melatonin and ramelteon are thought to promote a regular sleep cycle, although evidence for efficacy is uncertain in dementia. If a benzodiazepine is considered, lorazepam or oxazepam is preferred because they are shorter acting. These medications are summarized in Table 8.7. Side-effects to monitor include residual daytime sedation, worsening cognition, and gait disturbance.

★ TIPS AND TRICKS

If there is another symptom that is present, often a sedating medication used for that symptom can be dosed at bedtime to promote sleep as well. For example, the sedating antidepressant mirtazapine may be used to treat both depression and sleep disturbance. If a patient has agitation or psychosis, quetiapine is an atypical antipsychotic medication whose sedating effects may also help with sleep.

Depression

Depression in dementia can be difficult to assess, in part because other diagnoses or situations can be mistaken for depression, and vice versa. For example, patients with early dementia can appear depressed but may actually be undergoing a normal adjustment to the diagnosis of this disabling and fatal illness, or they are mourning the loss of their abilities and relationships. On the other hand, some patients with significant depression can be missed if normal adjustment or mourning is assumed in all cases. In later dementia stages, caregivers or healthcare providers may suspect depression in patients who appear sad and less interactive, but the patients themselves cannot verbally confirm that they have a depressed mood.

Table 8.7 Medications for sleep disturbance

Medication	Dose (mg at bedtime)
Trazodone	25–100
Zolpidem	5–10
Zaleplon	5–10
Eszopiclone	1–3
Melatonin	1–2
Ramelteon	8
Lorazepam	0.5–1
Oxazepam	7.5–15

Some criteria do exist to help with diagnosis. The DSM-5 criteria for Major Depressive Disorder requires five of the following for 2 weeks, where at least one is depressed mood or loss of interest: (1) depressed mood, (2) loss of interest or diminished pleasure, (3) appetite change, (4) sleep disturbance, (5) psychomotor changes (agitation or retardation), (6) fatigue, (7) worthlessness or guilt, (8) impaired concentration, or (9) thoughts of death. Provisional depression of AD criteria have been proposed, which modify Major Depressive Disorder criteria by reducing required elements to three (instead of five), removing impaired concentration, adding irritability, and separating loss of interest into two criteria (social withdrawal and decreased positive affect).

Although diagnosing depression in dementia can be challenging, there are two dementia types in which depression has a prominent role and where it may be wise to err towards a depression diagnosis. In Parkinson's disease, depression can predate and may be a prodrome for motor symptoms. Depression can continue to be a clinically significant concern even in later stages when PDD emerges. With vascular dementia where cerebrovascular accidents have recently occurred, there is an increased possibility of emerging depression. Poststroke depression is increasingly being recognized as having a negative impact on rehabilitation and quality of life, and therefore warrants treatment.

Treatment involves non-pharmacological and pharmacological approaches. Positive activities, such as those offered in adult day healthcare centers or in structured programs at long-term care facilities, can improve depressed mood in many patients. Treatment guidelines also recommend a trial of an antidepressant when depression is persistent and clinically important. Those medications with more favorable side-effects profiles in elderly patients include the SSRIs, serotonin norepinephrine reuptake inhibitors, and mirtazapine (see Tables 8.2 and 8.3).

EVIDENCE AT A GLANCE

The evidence supporting antidepressant use for depression in dementia is mixed at best, and the inclusion of antidepressant treatment in guidelines has been questioned. Examples include the DIADS-2 study, which investigated the antidepressant sertraline, and the HTA-SADD study, which investigated sertraline and mirtazapine. Researchers found improvement in most participants, including those taking placebo, such that there was no difference between active drug and placebo groups. However, side-effects were more common in those taking active drug.

Of the SSRIs, citalopram and sertraline are preferred because of fewer drug–drug interactions which may be of concern in medically complex and frail patients. Side-effects are generally mild. Rare but serious adverse effects to monitor include gastrointestinal bleeding and hyponatremia. The maximum dose of citalopram was reduced by the FDA due to a dose-related effect on prolonging the QTc interval. The serotonin norepinephrine reuptake inhibitor venlafaxine is also a good antidepressant choice, especially if a patient does not initially respond to an SSRI. Mirtazapine's sedating properties may be useful in patients with concomitant sleep disturbance.

Apathy

It is important to differentiate apathy from depression, as apathy is a distinctly different clinical syndrome. Rather than a mood state, apathy is primarily a decreased ability to initiate activities. Patients will have decreased motivation, reduced goal-directed behavior and cognitive activity, and worsened social disengagement. Apathy can be a considerable source of distress to caregivers as they see their loved ones gradually stopping involvement in previous activities.

Even though patients are less able to initiate activity, most still enjoy activities if the initiating steps are done for them. For example, caregivers can bring patients to events even when patients do not appear initially interested. Structured or organized activities, such as those offered in adult day health programs or senior centers, can also improve quality of life in patients with apathy.

The class of medications with the best evidence for efficacy is the cholinesterase inhibitors. Therefore it is important to consider a trial if a patient has not yet started one. There is some evidence that memantine may be useful as well. The stimulant drug methylphenidate may be useful for patients whose apathy interferes with necessary care. If prescribing methylphenidate, dosing starts at 2.5 mg twice daily, increasing by 2.5–5 mg as needed to a maximum of 10 mg twice daily.

Behavioral-variant frontotemporal dementia

Behavioral-variant frontotemporal dementia (bvFTD) is discussed separately here because the presentation and progression of bvFTD are different from other dementias. This disorder is characterized by the presence of severe behavioral symptoms very early in the clinical course, and behavioral symptoms are often noticed prior to cognitive impairment. It is not uncommon for bvFTD patients to initially be referred to psychiatrists because they are suspected of having a primary psychiatric condition rather than this rare neurodegenerative disease.

Patients are classically thought to have either a predominant apathy state or disinhibition, although many have both at some point in their disease course. Apathy can be profound, where the patient appears to lack empathy with others and loses motivation. Disinhibition can include hyperactive, hypersexual, and hyperoral behaviors. Stereotyped behaviors, such as repetitive clapping or what appear to be obsessive rituals, can also occur.

While the underlying pathophysiology is not fully understood, there may be a deficiency in serotonin with a relatively intact cholinergic system. Consistent with this, there is limited but suggestive evidence that SSRIs and trazodone may reduce behavioral symptoms (see Tables 8.2 and 8.3). Cholinesterase inhibitors may worsen behaviors in bvFTD, so they are best avoided. It is uncertain whether antipsychotic medications or anticonvulsants are helpful in bvFTD.

Further reading

Banerjee S, Hellier J, Dewey M, et al. Sertraline or mirtazapine for depression in dementia (HTA-SADD): a randomized, multicentre, double-blind, placebo-controlled trial. *Lancet* 2011; **378**: 403–11.

Berman K, Brodaty H, Withall A, et al. Pharmacologic treatment of apathy in dementia. *Am J Geriatr Psychiatry* 2012; **20**: 104–22.

Huey ED, Putnam KT, Grafman J. A systematic review of neurotransmitter deficits and treatments in frontotemporal dementia. *Neurology* 2006; **66**: 17–22.

Peskind ER, Tsuang DW, Bonner LT, et al. Propranolol for disruptive behaviors in nursing home residents with probable or possible Alzheimer disease: a placebo-controlled study. *Alzheimer Dis Assoc Disord* 2005; **19**: 23–8.

Rabins PV, Blacker D, Rovner BW, et al. American Psychiatric Association practice guideline for the treatment of patients with Alzheimer's disease and other dementias. Second edition. *Am J Psychiatry* 2007; **164**(12 Suppl): 5–56.

Raskind MA, Barnes RF. Alzheimer's disease: treatment of noncognitive behavioral abnormalities. In: Davis K, Charney D, Coyle J, Nemeroff C (eds) *Psychopharmacology: The Fifth Generation of Progress*. New York: Lippincott Williams and Wilkins, 2002, pp1253–65.

Rodda J, Morgan S, Walker Z. Are cholinesterase inhibitors effective in the management of the behavioral and psychological symptoms of dementia in Alzheimer's disease? A systematic review of randomized, placebo-controlled trials of donepezil, rivastigmine and galantamine. *Int Psychogeriatr* 2009; **21**: 813–24.

Rosenberg PB, Drye LT, Martin BK, et al. Sertraline for the treatment of depression in Alzheimer disease. *Am J Geriatr Psychiatry* 2010; **18**: 136–45.

Salami O, Lyketsos C, Rao V. Treatment of sleep disturbance in Alzheimer's dementia. *Int J Geriatr Psychiatry* 2011; **26**: 771–82.

Schneider LS, Tariot PN, Dagerman KS, et al. Effectiveness of atypical antipsychotic drugs in patients with Alzheimer's disease. *N Engl J Med* 2006; **355**: 1525–38.

Seitz DP, Adunuri N, Gill SS, et al. Antidepressants for agitation and psychosis in dementia. *Cochrane Database Syst Rev* 2011; **2**: CD008191.

Wang LY, Shofer JB, Rohde K, et al. Prazosin for the treatment of behavioral symptoms in patients with Alzheimer disease with agitation and aggression. *Am J Geriatr Psychiatry* 2009; **17**: 744–51.

9

Palliative Care in Advanced Dementias

Ira Byock[1] and Cory Ingram[2]

[1] Dartmouth-Hitchcock Medical Center, USA
[2] Mayo Clinic, College of Medicine, Mayo Clinic Health System, USA

Introduction and overview

Dementias are clinical syndromes caused by various diseases of the central nervous system and characterized by acquired persistent functional decline and intellectual impairments including, but not limited to, memory, executive function, language, and visual spatial skills. Alzheimer's type dementia is the most common primary form of dementia[1]. It is a terminal condition with no treatments currently available to cure or reverse the pathophysiology of the disease. In the United States, there are an estimated 5 million people who have Alzheimer's disease and this number is predicted to increase to 8 million by 2030. It is the fifth leading cause of death among American adults. Recent data from the Centers for Disease Control and Prevention demonstrate that deaths from Alzheimer's disease rose by 33% from 2000 to 2004 during which time deaths from heart disease, cerebrovascular disease, and many malignancies declined. The incidence of dementia of all causes rises by age. Approximately a third of all people over 85 years old may meet criteria for the diagnosis of dementia[2] and as many as one half have at least a mild impairment of memory and cognition.

> ### ✋ CAUTION
>
> Dementia is most common in the geriatric population. A list of medications called the Beers Criteria for Potentially Inappropriate Medication Use in Older Adults identifies common medications with a heightened risk of

causing adverse effects in elderly patients, particularly those with dementia[19]. Careful consideration should be given before continuing or initiating a medication on the Beers List in dementia patients.

One specific subset of Beers List medications[21], both prescribed and over the counter, known to have anticholinergic side-effects can compromise personal safety by causing worsening confusion and increased falls in patients with dementia. Commonly used anticholinergic medications to be avoided are diphenhydramine available over the counter and used for sleep, amitriptyline for depression, and oxybutinin for urge incontinence.

Because it is a disease of older adults, people with dementia often have co-existing chronic illnesses of various degrees that affect their digestive tracts, hearts, lungs, kidneys, livers, marrow and blood, spine, hands, feet and joints, eyes, and ears. This results in a significant symptom burden and clinical challenge to effectively assess and treat a person's discomforts and distress. Clinicians must assess atypical presentations within a frequently complex landscape of co-morbidities and changing baseline of function and cognitive capacity. A wise clinician draws on the observations of nurses and other professionals and family caregivers in making assessments. Whenever a patient's distress is severe or

Dementia, First Edition. Edited by Joseph F. Quinn.
© 2014 John Wiley & Sons, Ltd. Published 2014 by John Wiley & Sons, Ltd.

prolonged, evaluation and direct examination of the patient by a doctor are essential.

Dementias are rightly considered to be terminal conditions. Whether as a distinct progressive disease (such as Alzheimer's or Pick's) or in combination with other co-morbidities (as in the case of vascular dementia), dementias contribute to shortening affected people's lives. In one Dutch study, only 14% of people with dementia survived to an advanced to late stage dementia[3].

Despite the prevalence of severe cognitive impairments, the health system does not always serve patients with dementia well. An example is a recent study finding that 19% of nursing home decedents with cognitive issues had at least one burdensome transition of care near the end of life. Burdensome transitions were defined as those that "occurred in the last 3 days of life, if there was a lack of continuity in nursing homes after hospitalization in the last 90 days of life, or if there were multiple hospitalizations in the last 90 days of life[4]." Nursing home residents in regions with the highest quintile of such transitions were significantly more likely to have a feeding tube, spend time in an intensive care unit (ICU) in the last month of life, have stage IV decubitus ulcer or have late enrollment in a hospice. Clearly, some of the suffering that people with dementia experience through the end of life is based in systems rather than the disease and should be amenable to systemic quality improvements.

Predictable patient and family needs – and essential elements of dementia care

From the moment the diagnosis is made, or even suspected, affected individuals and their families have several predictable needs. They need access to information and if it is not available in the doctor's office, they need to be referred to sources of reliable information, which may include advice regarding credible online resources. People need support in adjusting to the current and future implications of the illness. Support in this context means more than a compassionate ear. Supportive counseling often entails significant time invested in understanding the particular details of people's lives, values and perspectives, so that professional caregivers can help them understand the impact of the diagnosis and functional prognosis on the person's or family's living situations, plans, hopes, and fears.

From the beginning of the illness, it is important to involve patients and their families in an ongoing process of education about their condition and shared decision making to identify patient-centered medical goals and plan for predictable medical decisions and contingencies. This includes having specific crisis management plans.

Such counseling and care planning are central to good care for patients with dementia. Clinicians caring for dementia patients are encouraged to discuss a full range of topics that affect a patient's physical and emotional well-being. However, at a minimum, physician–patient or family education and care planning must include whether or not to institute potentially life-prolonging treatments, including cardiopulmonary resuscitation, mechanical ventilation, kidney dialysis, and medically administered nutrition and hydration. When trials of life-prolonging treatments are desired, it is helpful for physicians to prospectively discuss patients' and families' thoughts about when or under what circumstances the treatments could be withdrawn.

Additionally, family members and friends who are, or will soon be, caregivers need training and practical support, as well as information, tips, and resources for their own health and well-being. It sounds reasonable and straightforward, but these basic services are not always readily available and such needs may go unmet, resulting in unnecessary pain, strain, confusion, and suffering on the part of both patients and those who love them.

Specialist palliative care teams are increasingly available within hospitals, long-term care, and community healthcare agencies to assist in addressing the needs of both patients and families. Palliative care teams extend practical assistance in navigating health systems and coordinating care, as well as responding to patients' physical, emotional, spiritual, and social distress and striving to enhance the quality of their daily lives. Hospice is the most familiar form of palliative care. Hospice programs deliver interdisciplinary team-based care to people who are dying, including the late stages of dementia. Hospice has been shown to benefit both patients and families[5]. Hospice services are typically available to support families in caring for patients in their homes, but a hospice can also serve patients in long-term care settings in conjunction with facility staff.

In contemporary healthcare, medical services are intentionally problem based. Health services respond to core health problems of injuries and diseases. The corresponding goals of problem-based medicine are to cure, prolong life, and restore function. These goals determine how clinicians assess patients and develop treatment plans. In the context of patients with dementia, often with significant co-morbid conditions, curing and restoring function are out of reach and alleviating suffering and enhancing quality of life become paramount goals. Since death is inevitable, at some point the best care must extend beyond cure or maximizing function to ensuring a safe and comfortable dying experience. In caring for people facing the end of life, more medical treatment does not always represent better care.

This chapter outlines a practical palliative care approach to caring for people with dementia and their informal caregiving network of family and friends. Our "Watch Over Me" approach is offered as a guide for neurologists, as well as non-neurological clinicians, students, and allied professionals of many disciplines in framing and planning care for dementia patients and their families (http://coryingrammd.com/file/Watch_Over_Me.html). The approach is based in trust and responsive to the affected person's and family's individual values, priorities and preferences, fears, and hopes. It extends to communication with patients and their families in the process of shared decision making, care planning, and anticipatory guidance for life completion and closure.

CASE

Mrs J is a 79-year-old widow who presented to our regional medical center through the emergency department and is now in the ICU. It is her fifth hospitalization in the last 6 months. Each time, she is transported by ambulance from a nursing home for evaluation of a fever, agitation, and possible stroke. This time the ambulance was called for respiratory distress. Recurrent evaluations during recent hospitalizations have included computed tomography (CT) and magnetic resonance imaging (MRI) scans of her head, chest, and abdomen. In each instance, by the time the acute problems were resolved, they were attributed to aspiration pneumonitis. During an admission 6 weeks ago, a percutaneous

gastric feeding tube was placed to supplement her nutrition and in hopes of preventing further aspiration.

For over 2 years, she has been unable to consistently recognize her family. For the last 9 months she has been dependent on others for bathing, dressing, and eating. She no longer has control over her bowel and bladder functions. She requires assistance by two nurses to transfer from bed to chair in the nursing facility.

Over the past 5 years Mrs J has been in four different nursing facilities, changing facilities twice in the last 6 months. Now she is intubated, sedated and on pressure support ventilation in the ICU. As you enter the room, you recognize Sally, one of her four children, whom you met during a previous admission. Sally sits at her mother's bedside with her head in her hands. She looks up and acknowledges you, dries her eyes, and gently drapes a rosary around her mother's limp left hand.

"Here we are again," she says to you, her half-smile and tone of voice apologetic. "I got a call from the nursing home that Mom was coughing and had trouble breathing. I didn't know what else to do. I talked with my sister and brothers. We're just not ready to 'pull the plug.'"

Disease trajectory, dementia treatment, and prognosis

On average, persons with Alzheimer's disease have a life expectancy of 8–10 years after diagnosis. The disease trajectory charts a jagged arc of predictable but often stuttering decline, commonly characterized by episodes of acute illness resulting in functional worsening and most often a recovery to a new, lower baseline. Prognosis in these conditions pertains not only to life expectancy but also to prospects for both future functional capacity and caregiving needs. Common life-altering illnesses for people with dementia are infections of the respiratory and genitourinary tracts, in addition to falls with fractures, commonly of the humerus, pelvis or hips. In far-advanced stages of dementia, some people lose interest in eating and drinking and may even push away a spoon or cup. Injuries and changes of this nature often herald the final phase of a dementia patient's life.

Treatments to maintain cognitive function or slow disease progression, such as cholinesterase inhibitors and N-methyl-D-aspartate (NMDA) receptor antagonists, have been addressed in earlier chapters of this volume. Clinical science has yet to answer the question of when or under what circumstances such medications should be withdrawn because they will yield little or no benefit, even if they are not causing adverse effects. In dire situations such as the ICU scenario of "Mrs J", most clinicians and caregivers would agree that there is no value to continuing such medications. Expert consensus would suggest that these medications are unlikely to improve the condition of bedbound, otherwise dependent, non-verbal patients in any meaningful way. In earlier stages of dementia, when there are valuable functions to maintain, such as recognizing family or being able to interact, and assisting in self-care, most clinicians recommend, and most patients and families agree, that if such medications are well tolerated, they are worth continuing.

Patients who have recently been diagnosed with dementia, particularly those in the early stage of progressive dementia, and their families commonly seek treatments for the disease. Early on, they are discouraged to discover the paucity of disease-modifying options currently available. Patients and families require education to adjust to the new reality of the diagnosis as well as to anticipate coming changes and plan for the future. Plans of care must respond to a patient's and family's current needs and strive to avoid crises along the way. Comprehensive care for patients with dementia and their families includes skillful support for making medical decisions in ways consistent with their personal values and preferences.

Whole-person and family-centered care encompasses assisting people in achieving a sense of life completion and closure, including, if they so choose, leaving a personal legacy, fulfilling individual and family values, roles and responsibilities to one another, and fostering a sense of celebration for the affected person and their family.

⬡ SCIENCE REVISITED

Delirium is a condition patients with dementia are more prone to experience. Often delirium is underrecognized and clinically the patient and family may be told that the dementia is rapidly worsening. This is incorrect, but understandable because delirium is an acute alteration of cognition hallmarked by disorganized thinking and inattention. The message to the family is that their loved one with dementia now has a condition called delirium that acutely and likely temporarily has worsened their abilities to function as they knew them just a few days ago. It is a condition that has many causes: infection, pain, medication, and electrolyte abnormalities. The delirium is likely to clear in the days, weeks, and months to come. There is a chance that their loved one will not regain their predelirium functional status.

The clinician can use the CAM-ICU test at the bedside to test for inattentiveness and disorganized thinking. The test is quick, easy, and inexpensive. The development of delirium is associated with an increased risk of mortality. This may be a good opportunity to revisit goals of care and advance care planning with the patient and family.

Alleviating suffering and improving quality of life

Alleviation of suffering and improving quality of life are key goals in caring for people with advanced dementia – and they are core goals for the discipline of palliative care.

Patients with dementia are at high risk of receiving inadequate assessments and treatment for physical discomfort. Evaluating pain and other physical distress in a patient with advanced dementia can be difficult. The limitations of cognition and communication must be approached by the clinical team in a systematic fashion. The pathogenesis of dementia typically does not alter pain pathways. However, neurodegenerative changes of dementia commonly affect people's perception of pain and their affective responses. Patients may not be able to localize pain, verbally describe or otherwise express their discomfort. A targeted physical examination is often necessary to uncover the location and cause of physical distress.

Self-reporting is the gold standard for documenting the frequency and rating the severity of pain, but because self-reports may be inconsistent, incongruent with clinical observations, or simply unfeasible in patients with dementia, behavioral and observational criteria have been developed. The Checklist of Non-verbal Pain Indicators takes nonverbal vocalizations, grimacing, wincing, bracing, rubbing, restlessness, and vocal complaints into consideration[6].

Patients with dementia may also demonstrate particular clinical patterns that represent their own individualized pain or physical discomfort signature. Such patterns may include withdrawal from social activities, agitation, wandering, insomnia, and stopping eating. Sometimes patients with even mild-to-moderate dementia will only exhibit signs of distress, irritability or agitation and be found to have a urinary infection, compression fracture, toothache, or zoster. Arthritis or degenerative joint disease is the most common source of pain in people with dementia.

Optimal management of pain and other physical distress typically depends on elucidating the etiology of the symptoms. That being said, there are a few caveats and things to keep in mind in treating pain in patients with dementia. Acetaminophen can be safely used in doses less than 4 g per day in most elderly patients, and 3 g a day in those with mild-to-moderate liver disease. A therapeutic trial of acetaminophen may be useful to see if it improves mood or behavioral signs of discomfort. Non-steroidal antiinflammatory medications carry the risk of both gastric and duodenal ulceration and renal compromise. Opioids have no tissue toxicity and may be used safely if dosed according to basic guidelines and principles of opioid prescribing. Opioid-naive patients with advanced dementia can be started on scheduled, low-dose short-acting opioids given by mouth. *Pro re nata* (prn) medications are difficult to use due to limitations of self-reporting. However, in settings such as special memory loss units, prn medications can be used based on serial observations by experienced nurses and other direct care staff. Side-effects commonly include constipation, which must be treated with laxatives, and transient, mild worsening of confusion to which most patients will accommodate over time.

Palliative care approaches dying as a difficult but normal stage and process of life[7] and extends the concept of quality of life to a person's dying experience. In addition to treating pain and associated bodily discomfort, palliative care strives to improve quality of life for patients and caregivers. Quality of life is inherently subjective. Simply put, it is how a person feels. Quality of life can be thought of as ranging on a linear scale from distress, suffering, and even agony, at one pole, to comfort, contentment, and joy at the other. Early in the course of progressive dementia, a patient may be able to express their quality of life, while in later stages, the assessment of quality of life usually turns on the observations of family members, lay caregivers, or professionals.

The perceived quality of a person's life informs decision making related to medical treatments and to the choice of supported living arrangements

Activities of daily living and dementia staging simplified

The tasks of navigating our days and world have been aptly divided into activities of daily living (ADL) and instrumental activities of daily living (iADL) and a checklist or inventory of ADLs and IADLs is essential when staging dementia. A simple approach to remembering the difference is to think of ADLs as everything you do in the morning to prepare yourself for the day, such as bathing, dressing, transferring, toileting, grooming, and feeding yourself. IADLs are everything you do after you are ready for the day to navigate the world, such as managing finances, transportation, medication, communications, laundry, house work, shopping, and cooking.

Reisberg defined seven stages of dementia[8]. As with the inventory of ADLs and IADLs, the simplification of a range of conditions into stages can be useful in understanding patients' experience, anticipating and preparing for pertinent issues and problems. In stage I, there are no clinical symptoms. Stage II is characterized by a person complaining about forgetfulness. In stage III other people typically begin to notice a person's functional deficits. A hallmark of stage IV is the impairment of one or several IADLs with preservation of ADLs. Because of disorientation and progressive loss of IADLs, stage V is often described by the saying "All dressed up and nowhere to go." People in stage V appear well dressed and ready for the day but they are disoriented and unable to perform most IADL's – hence, all dressed up and nowhere to go. Stage VI is marked by incontinence, an inability to recognize loved ones, and wandering.

It can be thought of as the "Velcro" stage in which people tend to cling to others, particularly in dementia facilities or nursing homes. In stage VII a person is dependent in ADLs and can only speak a few words. They are dependent on others for mobility such as rotation in bed and transfer for toileting and wheelchair. Most time is spent in bed unable to effectively communicate with others.

End-of-life care in dementia can be thought of as spanning stages V, VI, and VII, and may progress over many months or several years. In stage VII patients are dependent in ADLs and clearly approaching the end of their lives. Unfortunately, at present only in the later sub stages of stage VII, when the affected person is unable to ambulate or speak more than six words in a day, are patients with dementia eligible to receive hospice care under current Medicare criteria.

Families' journeys and supportive counseling

Whenever one person receives a serious diagnosis, a family experiences the subsequent illness. A core principle of palliative care sees each patient's family as part of the unit of care. Virtually every patient with advanced dementia has a family, whether by blood, marriage, or friendship. For an elderly person with advanced dementia, family can be expressed by the phrase, "for whom the person matters." Operationally, a frail person's family encompasses the people who visit, call and physically care for the person, which often includes long-time nurses, aides, and housekeepers.

Physicians and clinical teams can support each family member and guide a cohesive process of making decisions and providing care. Children, parents or siblings of the person with dementia can be expected to have discernible styles of relating to one another – and making decisions – that have been formed by their personal histories and family culture. An understanding of the family system can help in counseling patients and family members in coping and caregiving throughout the illness. The dominant personalities and decisional style of a family often become apparent over time. There may be *insiders* and *outsiders* in a family's patterns of conversing, making decisions, or providing care. Distance, time, and financial resources may all contribute, but a family's history and its members'

personalities also shape the ways in which people approach these difficult situations. Clinicians can astutely take note of these family characteristics, without judging which members of a divided family are right or wrong. Observations of a family's style, which may vary by ethnic culture, are valuable in counseling people who are struggling not only with treatment decisions, but also with the physical, emotional, and social strains of a loved one's dementia. Skillful clinicians can identify sources of strength within families and guide members in coming to agreement and, correspondingly, avoiding conflict.

Having someone they love become seriously ill naturally makes people feel emotionally vulnerable; it evokes worry, anxiety, and fears. Supportive counseling for a family member of a patient with advanced dementia can start by "stating the obvious." We have found that this puts family members (including a patient's close friends) at ease and builds a therapeutic alliance to say aloud that it is apparent how much they love and are worried about the person who is our patient.

Similarly, during family meetings for the sake of making decisions, when differences of opinion are voiced – or tempers flare – between family members, it is often helpful to explicitly acknowledge that despite disagreements, everyone present loves the person who is ill and therefore, everyone present is hurting. Clinicians can add that people come at these decisions differently – and we may or may not be able to come to an agreement about whether and for how long to use specific treatments – but each one is trying to do what they consider right and best for the person.

A family's journey – from prediagnosis, through the diagnosis, early treatments, corresponding changes in personal plans and shifts in roles, through chronic care, shared care, institutionalized care, and ultimately through the end of life and into grief – will be as unique as a fingerprint. Yet within the singular, personal experiences of every patient and family there are predictable challenges, decisions, and dynamics that every family is likely to encounter.

When an elderly mother or father becomes affected with dementia, adult children commonly feel conflicted about making decisions, sometimes against the parent's wishes. Common examples are a decision to no longer allow the person to drive, use the stove or a credit card.

We have found it helpful to present these challenges as developmental stages within the lifecycle of a family. During adolescence, parents often need to enforce limits for the safety and well-being of the teenager, even when it makes the young person angry and causes a scene. To do otherwise would be irresponsible. When dementia robs a parent of the ability to safely drive or use a stove top, it is only responsible for the children, who were once those teenagers, to set limits, even if doing so makes their mother or father angry – and causes a scene. Most families eventually come to realize this on their own, but anticipatory guidance by a clinician can facilitate the process, avoiding a lot of confusion and guilty feelings along the way.

Decision making and advance care planning

Individuals who engage in advance care planning (ACP) are likely to see several specific benefits for themselves and their loved ones. The person with dementia is more likely to have their end-of-life desires known and followed. They experience a better quality of life and endure fewer invasive procedures and fewer ICU admissions at the end of life. Their family experiences less stress and more satisfaction. The costs of their care – to families as well as Medicare – are correspondingly less. Advance directives have been shown to decrease family conflict and distress, be associated with fewer transfers to hospitals, less death in hospitals and in ICUs, less use of cardiopulmonary resuscitation (CPR) and mechanical ventilation before death, and a higher likelihood that personal end-of-life wishes will be honored. Whenever possible, advance care planning should include the completion of formal advance directive documents. These documents can be emotionally challenging for patients and families to complete, but they can provide family members with clear authority to make decisions for their loved ones and, by clearly conveying the individual's wishes, can alleviate the burden that families may feel in making decisions during future, life-threatening complications of the illness. Care planning that involves patients and their families in collaboration with the patients' physicians and clinical teams is an ongoing process.

★ TIPS AND TRICKS

The Physician's Order for Life Sustaining Treatment (POLST) is a document that the patient and physician review and complete, clearly stating what treatments the patient would want in life-threatening conditions. The POLST translates the individual preferences of a patient or legal surrogate into formal physician (or other authorized clinician) orders related to performance or avoidance of CPR, mechanical ventilation, renal dialysis, provision of medically administered nutrition and hydration, and transfers to a hospital. Medical interventions may be tailored to the person's preferences to include full invasive care, comfort measures only and itemization of treatments that fall in the middle to include intravenous fluids, antibiotics, and less invasive airway support. In contrast to an advance directive, the POLST document provides emergency personnel with clear, real-time orders in crisis situations. The POLST is an important tool for honoring patients' wishes, providing care in accordance with discussions with patients or their chosen decision makers, and preventing conflicts.

Counseling and anticipatory guidance for advanced stage dependence

In approaching patients' and families' experiences of dementia as a difficult stage of life with predictable challenges, clinicians can provide anticipatory guidance for the decisions, dangers, and opportunities that lie ahead. The concept of anticipatory guidance is drawn from pediatrics, in which clinicians not merely attend to medical problems but also preserve opportunities for patients and families to grow individually and together through developmental stages.

In the context of the trajectory of a person's dementia, anticipatory guidance may encompass advice and education designed to prevent problems and foster well-being, in situations that carry significant risk of physical and emotional distress.

Anticipatory guidance for the patient and family includes honestly taking stock of current levels of functioning and identifying signs of potential upcoming decline. It requires a respectful balance between independence and safety. Corresponding to the analogy of adolescence, adult children now tend to give more weight to safety, while the now elderly parent may vociferously declare their right to independence despite concerns for their welfare.

As dementia worsens, a creative, shared approach to ADLs can help maintain a balance between safety and independence. As with young children, the level of participation and requisite supervision should be proportionate to the person's capacity to understand and derive value from the experience. For instance, by stage IV of dementia, driving alone or at night may not be safe, but having a "co-pilot" may safely enable limited daytime driving. In stage V, people will have lost abilities to perform IADLs and will likely be dependent in grooming or other ADLs. They may not wander, but would certainly get lost in unfamiliar settings if left alone. People in stages IV and V are often able to express themselves and may be able to reminisce, tell favorite stories, celebrate special family events, including birthdays and holidays, as well as funerals.

Ultimately, as the disease advances and enters its late stages, people with dementia become fully dependent on others.

In later stages, it becomes essential to err on the side of safety in caring. In stages V and VI of a dementing illness, progressive incontinence, wandering, and progressive inability to recognize family members should prompt more explicit planning for the end of life. This is particularly true for patients with co-morbid conditions, as they are less likely to benefit from invasive therapies such as CPR, artificial hydration and nutrition, and ventilation.

In the absence of co-morbidities and acute complications, progressive dementia causes death principally through urinary or respiratory infections or malnutrition. Incontinence may force trade-offs between skin breakdown and the heightened risk of infection that accompanies an indwelling catheter. Difficulties with swallowing may force a choice between aspirating food and fluids, accepting gradual malnutrition, or pursuing low-yield treatments, including PEG tube nutrition and hydration.

Although interdisciplinary palliative care may be of value throughout the course of progressive dementia, specialized palliative care, including hospice care, should be provided to patients with stage VII dementia and their families.

Life completion and closure

As with other life-limiting conditions, people diagnosed with dementia often value an opportunity to feel complete in their personal affairs[9,10]. Life completion extends to responsibilities at work, to personal business and financial matters, as well as to personal relationships. Concrete tasks may include creating or updating a Last Will and Testament that delineates how one's possessions and estate are to be managed. An advance directive, such as Durable Power of Attorney for Health Care or a Living Will, authorizes one or more individuals to make medical decisions on behalf of the person, if they become incapacitated, and can provide guidance to the person who holds this responsibility. Both types of documents can lessen the burden that families feel, and may resolve disagreements and prevent (or lessen) family conflicts.

Like those who are facing the end of life, people who are entering a time of increasing physical dependence may be bothered by feeling that they are a burden to others and may value opportunities to contribute in some ways to friends and family. The exercises of life review, and telling and recording of one's life stories can be thought of as tasks which help to develop a sense of meaning about one's life and as a way of leaving a unique legacy to others[11]. Life review can enhance a person's sense of worth and dignity. Indeed, it forms a central part of dignity therapy for people approaching death[12]. For those diagnosed with progressive dementia, developmental tasks of life completion are often best supported as early as possible.

Watch Over Me: a framework and guiding principles for advanced dementia

"Watch Over Me" is the term we have applied to a set of guidelines which clinicians can use in providing practical support and counseling to patients with dementia and their families (http://coryingrammd. com/file/Watch_Over_Me.html). This framework is intended to address the needs and experiences of simultaneous trajectories of illness experienced by people with dementia and their caregivers. These experiences can be described through the stages of dementia for the person with the disease and corresponding stages in the family's journey. Each individual's and family's experiences are unique, yet these intentionally simplified schemas provide a context through which to address predictable problems and decisions regarding matters of physical health, living situation, and caregiver needs and well-being. Watch Over Me builds on trust between each patient and their caregivers, including the person's chosen proxy decision makers. It also builds on and fosters trust between a patient and family and the patient's doctor. Watch Over Me brings the trusting, covenantal values within loving relationships into the processes of planning and caring. It complements and balances the contractual values that are protective or defensive and are embedded in medical ethics and advance directives.

Communication with patients and families living with dementia is sometimes difficult and may be uncomfortable for physicians and other professional healthcare providers, yet it is always valued by patients and families and very often helpful in clarifying people's perspective and priorities, thereby informing current plans of care. How does a family express love, compassion, and the dedication to their loved one with advanced dementia? How does that family assure themselves and others that they are looking out for their loved one's best interests when at times they feel as though the decisions they are faced with leave their loved one without independence, dignity, and at the end of life without medical interventions to help them live? Is it possible to affirm an everlasting dedication to your loved one with dementia in the midst of difficult end-of-life decision making? Caregivers experience these thoughts and feelings, and they affect their well-being, decision making, and interactions with the healthcare teams. As a person with dementia progresses to stages V, VI and VII, life changes dramatically and certain crises become predictable, necessitating advance care planning. Communicating how the illness may play out informs professional and family caregivers how best to respond to the next crisis.

The basic framework and principles of advance care planning are consistent over time. Stated simply, it is a process of matching patient and family values and preferences to achievable health outcomes and personal goals[13]. Naturally, the specific topics discussed shift in response to the stage of illness. Treatment decisions that are confronting patients and/or their families and the treating clinicians change over time. Using the example of Mrs J, opportunities for supportive counseling, shared decision making and collaborative care planning change from

early stages and office settings, through later stages and residential care, through the acute hospitalizations and current ICU stay on mechanical ventilation.

Guiding principle #1: be prepared

It is best to prepare well for meetings with people such as Mrs J or her daughter, Sally. In addition to reviewing medical records from previous admissions, it is often useful to speak with previous clinicians and referring clinicians. The staff at a patient's memory unit or nursing facilities can provide invaluable descriptions of the person's recent baseline – their level of orientation, performance of IADLs and ADLs, continence, ambulation, and interactions with the family caregivers. Professional caregiving staff on specialized units often have a good understanding of functional milestones. The many interactions between family and professional caregivers will form lasting memories for the family about their loved one's dementia journey.

Guiding principle #2: create the space

Meetings with patients and families to discuss treatment options and make decisions are rightly seen as important medical procedures. It is therefore important to plan for such meetings and ensure that the key stakeholders and decision makers can participate. When a family member for whom it is important can't be present, they may be able to participate by phone or video conference call. In the case of Mrs J, we met her daughter Sally and the family in Mrs J's room in the ICU. We provided chairs for two of Sally's siblings and Sally's aunt who flew in to visit her sister. We also brought chairs for the medical staff attending the meeting.

Sitting down during the conversation with Sally, a family member who is worried and grieving, conveys the clinician's full attention to the conversation and the importance of the content to her mother. We got to know Mrs J's family and how they were related. The medical staff took turns explaining their role in Mrs J's care.

Guiding principle #3: set an agenda

In preparing and setting an agenda or set of topics for a meeting with a family whose loved one is seriously ill, clinicians can inquire what the family is hoping to achieve during and after the meeting. The facilitator can clarify the family's goals for the meeting and add goals identified by the medical staff.

Guiding principle #4: deliver the person with dementia from anonymity

It can be tempting to start to address the goals identified by the family and even offer information and solutions. However, the very act of holding a focused meeting of family and professional caregivers can serve as a therapeutic endeavor. In progressive diseases, a strictly problem-based approach to care may subtly conflict with a whole-person approach. Some problems cannot and will not be solved, but people can always be cared for and watched over. It is useful to reflect that family members are trying to watch over their loved one and that the foundations of decision making are based on love, trust, and times of reciprocal caregiving. It is a mistake to avoid "big picture" conversations by focusing immediately on decisions regarding feeding tubes, tracheostomies or long-term ventilation, or kidney dialysis. Doing so effectively depersonalizes the decision-making process and exiles doctors and families to islands of itemized medical problems and technological solutions. Arguably, this describes the decisional environment in the case of Mrs J; arguably, that environment and path led Mrs J to end up in the ICU.

In the case of Mrs J, a counseling strategy of inviting her, at least in spirit, to the conversation was key. It is essential, since she is the person around which the love, trust, and caregiving revolve. Knowledge of who she is as a person and the exploration of her life prior to dementia were not only therapeutic to Sally, but in coming to know her in this manner, the information gained and anecdotes collected informed the professional caregivers. In reviewing a patient's life with family members, clinicians will come to know who the person loves and who loves her, providing insights into the person's values in life, often enabling all involved to extrapolate to what they would value at this time of life.

For Mrs J to get the best care possible and for Sally to be supported by the medical professionals in making decisions for her mother, clinicians have to have talked about what Mrs J values. In our experience, the process of delivering non-verbal patients from anonymity, as coined by Dr Ned Cassem, joins the professional and family caregivers intellectually and emotionally as they embark on the most memorable conversations and crucial decisions they will make on a frail parent's behalf.

Guiding principle #5: state the obvious

Therapeutic responses to Sally can include recognition of the journey of her mother and of the family. Identify the balance between independence and safety that she navigated without a crisis despite the ambivalence and ambiguity she was experiencing. Name the guilt she must be feeling and enquire how she is coping.

Guiding principle #6: determine understanding of illness

It may seem rhetorical, after reviewing the chart, to request that caregivers itemize the medical problems their loved one is living with; however, this is an opportunity to ensure that you can pick up where their medical knowledge leaves off. Assuming that people know that dementia is a terminal disease can misguide clinicians in their conversations with family members. In our experience even family members of people with stage VI and VII dementia may not have been informed or understand that their loved one is in the latter stages of a disease that will cause death. It is prudent, therefore, to find out what caregivers and other family members understand. When necessary, it is important to explain explicitly that dementia – in combination with an itemized list of the person's major co-morbid conditions – will claim their loved one's life. This review of a person's problem list is not intended to emphasize all the problems to be solved, but more to create the context within which clinicians and families can explore realistic goals and redefine hope.

Guiding principle #7: identify hope

In a medical problem-based approach to end-of-life care, we often pair solutions with each problem on the list. However, the sum of all problem-based treatment plans does not result in a comprehensive patient- and family-centered plan of care. Within a strictly problem-based framework, as diseases progress and a person's physical and cognitive conditions deteriorate, all hope is lost.

Hope can be identified in several different ways, but we find it most simply in the conversation with Sally. After reviewing the current medical problems in common terms, the physician acknowledged how well Sally had done in very difficult times. He said: "I appreciate taking the time to review your mother's historical and current medical problems. You have a good understanding of your mother's very complex medical situation. It's fair to say that you and your mother have been through a lot. If it is OK with you, I'd like to ask a question that will help us know how we can best care for your mother. As we have discussed, your mother has declined in the last years. She now has stage VI dementia. And as you accurately said, her swallowing problems caused her to swallow some food into her lungs. That is what has caused the episodes of pneumonia. Now she is depending on a machine to breathe for her and she is not improving despite maximal medical care. As a result of how sick she is, her kidneys are not working and that has caused her to be less interactive and sleepier. Knowing this, Sally, it is unlikely that she is going to get well. I think we may have to adjust what we can hope for."

Any number of questions may come, and clarification may be needed, but often caregivers can clearly voice that they would like their loved one to die gently when the time comes. If that is the case then the problem list can be converted to a comfort care plan that honors the wish to die gently.

Sally was not able to let go of all hope that her mother would get stronger and be able to breathe on her own. But she also said that she didn't want her mother to suffer. At the end of the physician's conversation with Sally, they agreed to a time-limited trial of two additional days. He was able to say, "Whether or not your mother is physically better within a couple of days, we will make sure she is comfortable. I want to encourage and support you and your siblings and children to honor and celebrate her while she is here."

In the setting of non-acute care planning, understanding hope will help to inform whether patients will be (or remain) hospitalized with a limitless menu of medical interventions, or hospitalized with a limited, tailored menu of medical interventions, such as antibiotics, without intubation or CPR being allowed, or will not hospitalized but treated at home or in a long-term care facility with care directed to alleviating discomfort and distress and allowing them to die gently.

Guiding principle #8: normalize feelings of relief in grief

At times like these it can be therapeutic to acknowledge the sense of relief that most caregivers will feel when their loved one dies and the guilt they are feeling because they will be relieved.

Guiding principle #9: tailoring

Often when meeting with families of persons with dementia, there is difficulty in recognizing the burden of some treatments on patients with advanced dementia versus the benefit. It is often helpful to review and acknowledge the tailoring of their loved one's personal life and then enquire whether or not their medical life may similarly need to be tailored.

Guiding principle #10: everybody dies of something

When someone is diagnosed with one or more serious illnesses, often the worst thing people can imagine is that the person they love will die. In reality, however, clinicians know that even worse things are possible and that there is a risk that the person will die badly, suffering as they die, sometimes as a result of being treated in ways they would not have wanted.

It is important from the time of diagnosis to explain that conditions such as Alzheimer's disease are terminal illnesses, so that planning and decision making can occur in the context of a life-limiting condition. The principles within the Watch Over Me framework support a process of continuing to strive for the best care possible while acknowledging that optimal care must extend to the experience of dying.

As long as a person's quality of life is of value to them or to their family, treatments of infections and other reversible complications of illness should be considered. Decision making is often explained as striking a balance between risks and benefits. More precisely, decisions rest on the balance between known burdens of treatment combined with the risks or potential burdens of treatment, balanced against the potential benefits. This balancing occurs on a baseline quality of life that changes over time, tending to lean further away from invasive life-prolonging treatments as a person's functional capacity declines, IADLs and ADLS are progressively lost, and a person's quality of life may become less valuable to preserve. While not every person or family weighs decisions in this manner, many do.

These considerations apply during the processes of advance care planning and shared decision making in discussing with patients and families their feelings and preferences for how best to respond to fevers that signal potentially life-limiting infections and the progressive inability to eat and drink.

Treatment of infection makes sense early in the course of dementia, but infections may provide a natural and reasonably comfortable physiological way for people with advanced dementia to die. While medically administered nutrition and hydration are clearly life saving in situations when the cause of an inability to eat or drink can be corrected, in the course of progressive dementia, evidence strongly indicates that most people do not benefit from prolonged periods of tube nutrition. However, the issue of nutritional supplement carries profound symbolic power for families who may worry about "starving" their loved one to death. Families deserve substantial support to explore and understand the rationale of not placing a nasal or percutaneous feeding tube[14,15].

It seems logical and is tempting to extrapolate to frail patients with dementia the clear benefits of supplemental nutrition in malnourished patients prior to surgery or other definitive treatments for reversible conditions. The benefits people seek from artificial nutrition and hydration – reduced incidence of aspiration pneumonia and improved survival – have not been demonstrated in numerous studies. Studies do not demonstrate an increase in quality of life for patients with advanced dementia through medically administered hydration and nutrition.

By discussing CPR and mechanical ventilation in the context of Watch Over Me, family members msometimes come to understand that they are not "giving up" or choosing death, but rather choosing to allow the person to die gently rather than in the midst of a fight that ultimately is futile for all.

Often, in the United States, clinicians talk about goals of care for CPR and artificial nutrition and hydration with families whose loved ones have stage VII dementia. This is common in the hospital setting and upon admission to a long-term care facility. This practice is so endemic that even when well-documented advance directives or do not attempt resuscitation (DNAR) orders are on the chart, the patient and more often the caregiver are asked these questions. Daly reviewed the ethical and moral aspects of withholding CPR from patients who are unlikely to benefit[16].

Caregivers and family members of patients with advanced dementia are frequently asked about whether they want CPR performed if their loved one's heart were to stop. In our experience, it almost always makes people feel as though they are being asked to choose between life and death for the person they love. There is a disingenuous aspect to the question. In offering the therapy, CPR, there is an inherent suggestion that it may be of benefit to their loved one. During conversations with caregivers, we will often reframe the question. We suggest that the decision is really not one of life and death; instead, it is actually about whether their loved one will die with or without CPR. Will they die with CPR or be allowed to die peacefully? When surrogate decision makers see the journey that both the patient and family have completed in stage VII dementia, they are often able to express the hope of a gentle death for their loved one.

Guiding principle #11: goal-based versus problem-based approach to care: the unasked question

Medical care is often problem based. Due to the nature of late-stage dementia, these patients have medical problems that affect their eating, drinking, swallowing, speaking, walking, ability to get and clear infections, and freedom to die naturally. Commonly, patients with late-stage dementia and their families are asked to address each problem the patient is faced with. For example, if the person is not eating, the question of a feeding tube placement arises. If the person is suffering recurrent episodes of aspiration pneumonia, they are asked about swallowing studies and modified diet. If the person is being admitted to hospital, they are questioned about their wish to have CPR performed if their heart were to stop.

Science re-visited: Artificial hydration and nutrition

In a problem-based approach to caring for patients with dementia, consideration is often given to artificial hydration and nutrition through a tube, either NG or PEG, when the patient has developed stage VII dementia and is no longer eating, or perhaps in stage VI as a preventive measure for aspiration pneumonia. The evidence indicates that tube feedings are inadequate in preventing aspiration, worsen quality of life, and do not increase longevity in patients with dementia. Careful delineation of the goals of care is important when considering tube feeding for a patient with dementia[20,22].

Arguably, most interventions are burdensome and deliver little to no benefit to the patient with late-stage dementia. Due to the complex and often co-existing nature of multiple irreversible problems in a terminal disease such as dementia, one must ask questions related to the overall goals of care rather than the individual problems. In patients with dementia, questions about the goals of care can be embodied in what we refer to as "the unasked question." This is not about the itemized medical problems, but rather about the personal goals of the patient and family. It is called "unasked" because most often time and attention are spent on the problem-based approach and less on the goal-based approach. The unasked question is always a variation on a simple and meaningful personal theme; in very general terms, it is simply, "How do you envision your loved one's end of life playing out?" "How can we best care for them, knowing that your loved one is in the last stage of their terminal illness with serious complications that are unfortunately not amenable to treatments and interventions. Nature is providing them with natural ways of dying. If we intervene with a feeding tube, we are not making them immortal, but we are pushing their frail physical condition further so if they can't die from the natural way their disease is offering, what will they be allowed to die from?" In our experience, family members are wondering in the back of their minds how this will all play out for their loved one and when asked, they are usually receptive, relieved and understand the limited options they are facing as they watch over their loved one.

How then do you approach a conversation in which you want to ask a goal-based question to clarify how to care for someone in late-stage dementia? In palliative medicine, we recognize that patients and families want us to be sensitive to their willingness and preparedness to talk about serious illness and dying. The unasked question is one that cannot simply be asked without the proper context, trust, and conversational foundation. Therefore, the foundation of the conversation leading to the unasked question assumes we have given a warning shot of the seriousness of the situation, an acknowledgment of the difficulty the family are facing, and the opportunity to endorse our further pursuit of the more difficult issue at hand.

With this foundation and their permission, we often recount some of the disease journey and their loved one's progression over time. We honor their life. We acknowledge their family journey and commend them on their role in caring for their loved one. We honor their caregiving. We then just ask

something along these lines: "Given the fragile physical condition of your loved one, we can certainly do more for them, but we are not making them immortal. In fact, we are likely only to push their already fragile physical state even further, making them die of something even worse. Nature is giving them several natural ways to die peacefully. That being said, it appears the question at hand is what would it be OK for your loved one to die from if they can't die from this gentle way that nature provided for them? What would be an acceptable and comfortable way for your dear mother to die?"

Asking the unasked question allows professional and family caregivers to talk about how best to care for their loved one. A care plan can be made to honor the person's goals. This helps to understand what interventions are helpful to achieving the goals and not just their problems.

Watch Over Me: conversational guiding principles for advanced dementia

1) Honors the patient and family journey.
2) Contextualizes advance care planning and decision making based on both disease staging and the family journey.
3) Recognizes the patient's disease stage and provides anticipatory guidance.
4) Provides anticipatory guidance to form goals of care, allowing us to predict, prevent, and respond to crisis with a tailored care plan.
5) Therapeutically honors key family decision points based on ambiguity, ambivalence, independence, safety, and guilt.
6) Recognizes and supports families making end-of-life decisions, helping them to reframe hope and decision making more accurately so that decisions at the end of life are less between life and death and more about dying with or without particular interventions.
7) Normalizes the sense of relief most caregivers feel when their loved one with dementia dies.

Prognostication and hospice care in dementia

The National Hospice and Palliative Care Organization (NHPCO) hospice eligibility criteria have been set to allow only those people unfortunate enough to advance to stage VII dementia to enroll in hospice services. These criteria have a predictive value that a patient meeting them is likely in the last 6 months of life. As reviewed, stage VII is characterized by dependence in ADLs and an inability to communicate verbally. Hospice criteria also require a recent, last 12-month history of complicated recurrent genitourinary tract infections, aspiration pneumonia, stage 3 or 4 decubiti, septicemia, recurrent fevers, or 10% weight loss in the last 6 months or a serum albumin less than 2.5 g/dL[17]. It is easy to conclude that persons meeting hospice criteria have needed palliative care services for a long time, once again underscoring the role of palliative care in advance dementia.

The Mortality Risk Index (MRI) is a less frequently used alternative to the FAST stages as described by Reisberg[7] (Table 9.1). The MRI is a composite score based on 12 risk factor criteria obtained from using the minimum data set. It has greater predictive value of 6-month prognosis than the FAST. The MRI has only been evaluated in newly admitted nursing home residents[18].

Table 9.1 Mortality Risk Index

Points	Risk factor
1.9	Complete dependence with ADLs
1.9	Male gender
1.7	Cancer
1.6	Congestive heart failure
1.6	O_2 therapy needed w/in 14 days
1.5	Shortness of breath
1.5	Less than 25% of food eaten at most meals
1.5	Unstable medical condition
1.5	Bowel incontinence
1.5	Bedfast
1.4	Age >83 years
1.4	Not awake most of the day
Risk estimate of death within 6 months	
Score	Risk %
0	8.9
1–2	10.8
3–5	23.2
6–8	40.4
9–11	57.0
12	70.0

CASE CONTINUED

Mrs J: making the best of a difficult situation
Meeting Mrs J's daughter Sally in the ICU, her suffering seemed worse than her mother's. Mrs J was insensate, the result of sedatives required to maintain respiratory synchrony – and keep her from reflexively coughing against the ventilator.

I asked Sally to tell me about Mrs J as a person before this illness. In delivering her mother from anonymity, the atmosphere in the room changed, allowing Sally's mother to be present as a person in our minds and conversation. It let us honor her as a person. Even though I knew the medical history, I asked Sally to recount her mother's dementia history. She reflected on the ambivalence and ambiguity in the family at the time of her diagnosis. I took the opportunity to state the obvious and identify clear landmarks of the role change that had taken place in the family: the transition to chronic care, shared care, and institutionalized care as her mother currently lived in an assisted living memory unit. I reflected back to her that as a family, they had been through a lot. I commended her on avoiding crisis and making decisions in balancing independence and safety along the way. I paused to acknowledge the guilt that most family caregivers experience during this journey and she cried in affirmation.

Together, we recounted Mrs J's disease progression and staged the dementia as stage VI. Sally told me that in the hospital when they were asking her questions about CPR and feeding tubes, she had not even realized her mother had a terminal illness. We explored the characteristics of stage VI dementia and I provided anticipatory guidance as to what the future might look like. I reflected on the progression of hope and she confirmed that once she had hoped the doctors were wrong about the diagnosis. She had hoped that her mother would be cured. Hope then changed to "living as well as possible" with the disease and now she realizes that hope rests in her mother being well cared for and dying gently. Sally expressed the wish that her mother would die in her sleep. I suggested that CPR did not really have a role in dying gently and she agreed. Putting the family's journey into context and staging the disease allowed Sally to simply watch over her mother. The feeding tube topic followed in the same way. Simply stating the obvious, that most family members feel a sense of relief when their loved one dies, gave Sally permission to put into words feelings that she had been too insecure about to voice aloud. She thanked me and left with a care plan designed to anticipate the future, prevent and respond to predictable crises with advance care planning already made during a moment of reflection on her mother's and her own dementia journey, honoring and celebrating both during consultation.

Sally continues to watch over her mother.

Conclusion

Dementia will continue to represent a leading cause of death in our society and it will continue to cause suffering among patients and caregivers alike. Specialty palliative care consultant teams may be possible in some settings, but application of the palliative care principles reviewed in this chapter can serve practicing clinicians as they personalize care for patients living with dementia and their caregivers.

References

[1] Mendez MF, Cummings JL. *Dementia: A clinical approach*, 3rd edn. Philadelphia: Butterworth Heinemann, 2003.

[2] Koopmans R, van Weel C. Survival to late dementia in Dutch nursing home patients. *J Am Geriatr Soc* 2003; **51**(2): 184–7.

[3] Gozalo P, Teno JM, Mitchell SL, et al. End-of-life transitions among nursing home residents with cognitive issues. *N Engl J Med* 2011; **365**(13): 1212–21.

[4] Teno JM, Gozalo PL, Lee IC, et al. Does hospice improve quality of care for persons dying from dementia? *J Am Geriatr Soc* 2011; **59**(8): 1531–6.

[5] Nygaard HA, Jarland M. The Checklist of Nonverbal Pain Indicators (CNPI): testing of reliability and validity in Norwegian nursing homes. *Age Ageing* 2006; **35**(1): 79–81.

[6] Torke AM, Holtz LR, Hui S, et al. Palliative care for patients with dementia: a national survey. *J Am Geriatr Soc* 2010; **58**: 2114–21.

[7] Reisberg BG, Ferris SH, de Leon MJ, et al. The stage specific temporal course of Alzheimer's disease: functional and behavioral concomitants based upon cross-sectional and longitudinal observation. *Alzheimer's Dis Relat Disord* 1989; **317**: 23–41.

[8] Pattee J, Caron W, Otteson O. *Alzheimer's Disease: the family journey*. Plymouth, Maine: North Ridge Press, 2001.

[9] Caplan GA, Meller A, Squires B, Chan S, Willett W. Advance care planning and hospital in the nursing home. *Age and Ageing* 2006; **35**: 581–5.

[10] Byock I. The nature of suffering and the nature of opportunity at the end of life. *Clin Geriatr Med* 1996; **12**(2): 237–52.

[11] Steinhauser KE, Clipp EC, McNeilly M, Christakis NA, Tulsky JA. In search of a good death: observations of patients, families, and providers. *Ann Intern Med* 2000; **132**(10): 825–32.

[12] Steinhauser KE, Alexander SC, Byock IR, George LK, Tulsky JA. Seriously ill patients' discussions of preparation and life completion: an intervention to assist with transition at the end of life. *Palliat Support Care* 2009; **7**(4): 393–404.

[13] Chochinov HM. Dignity and the essence of medicine: the A, B, C, and D of dignity conserving care. *BMJ* 2007; **335**(7612): 184–7.

[14] Meier DE. Palliative care and the quality of life. *J Clin Oncol* 2001; **29**(20): 2750–2.

[15] Teno JM, Mitchell SL, Gozalo P, et al. Hospital characteristics associated with feeding tube placement in nursing home residents with advanced cognitive impairment. *JAMA* 2010; **303**(6): 544–50.

[16] Loeb MB, Becker M, Eady A, Walker-Dilks C. Interventions to prevent aspiration pneumonia in older adults: a systematic review. *J Am Geriatr Soc* 2003; **51**(7): 1018–22.

[17] Teno JM, Gozalo P, Mitchell S, et al. Terminal hospitalizations of nursing home residents: does facility increasing the rate of do not resuscitate orders reduce them? *J Pain Symptom Manage* 2011; **41**(6): 1040–7.

[18] Wenrich MD, Curtis JR Jr, Channon SE, et al. Comunicating with dying patients within the spectrum of medical care from terminal

diagnosis to death. *Arch Intern Med* 2001; **161**(6): 868–74.

[19] Schonwetter RS, Han B, Small BJ, et al. Predictors of six-month survival among patients with dementia: an evaluation of hospice Medicare guidelines. *Am J Hospice Palliat Care* 2003; **20**(2): 105–13.

[20] Mitchell SL, Kiely DK, Hamel MB, et al. Estimating prognosis for nursing home residents with advanced dementia. *JAMA* 2004; **291**: 2734–40.

[21] Beers Criteria Update Expert Panel. *J Am Geriatr Soc* 2012; **60**(4): 616–31.

[22] Finucane T, Bynum J. Use of tube feeding to prevent aspiration pneumonia. *Lancet* 1996; **348**: 1421–4.

10

Ethical, Legal, and Social Issues in Dementia

Amy Y. Tsou[1] and Jason Karlawish[2]

[1]Department of Neurology, Perelman School of Medicine at the University of Pennsylvania, USA
[2]Departments of Medicine and Medical Ethics, Perelman School of Medicine at the University of Pennsylvania, USA

Introduction

In ancient Greek mythology, the Lethe was one of five fabled rivers of the underworld, with powerful waters that washed away memory from those who had crossed over into the land of the dead. However, patients today with dementia and those who care for them must navigate the land of the living while memory slowly but inexorably ebbs away. Modern increases in life expectancy and a growing elderly population mean that an increasing number of patients and families will face the unique challenges of living with dementia. This chapter addresses these challenges' distinctive legal, social, and ethical features.

After describing the challenges, we review the principles medical ethics offers for considering decision making in patients with and without cognitive impairment. Next, we apply these principles to six practical problems. We conclude with reflections regarding dementia's broader social and cultural ramifications.

Distinctive aspects of providing care in dementia

The ability to make a choice has been considered foundational to many aspects of modern society and much of modern medical ethics has centered on efforts to promote and preserve patient autonomy. Autonomy means self-governance (*autos* "self" and *nomos* "rule, governance or law"). However, the characteristic memory loss and other cognitive impairments in dementia lead to gradual diminishment of both "self" and consequently "governance." As a result, decision-making paradigms built primarily around autonomous individual decision making by patients are inadequate.

Instead, caring for dementia patients requires a thoughtful approach to gauging the severity of cognitive dysfunction and whether or not these impairments diminish decision-making capacity. Furthermore, dementia care is distinguished not only by the loss of cognitive abilities, but the pace and tempo of decline. Unlike processes such as stroke or trauma in which cognitive abilities can be dramatically and quickly altered, progressive cognitive decline in dementia is typically quite gradual and, at times, even insidious. This incremental pace of decline requires clinicians and family members to remain engaged in an iterative process with repeated assessments of cognitive dysfunction, resultant decision-making capacity, and surveillance for new difficulties on the horizon. Given the many uncertainties surrounding disease progression, for the clinician, a significant component of caring for dementia patients and their families is active engagement in managing expectations and anxiety.

With disease progression, as patients fall silent, caregivers play an increasingly pivotal role in patient care. Much has been made of the privileged relationship that exists between doctors and patients. However, in dementia, this relationship necessarily

Dementia, First Edition. Edited by Joseph F. Quinn.
© 2014 John Wiley & Sons, Ltd. Published 2014 by John Wiley & Sons, Ltd.

broadens to include the caregiver(s). Not only are caregivers vital in maintaining the quality of care patients receive, but as patients become unable to decide for themselves, caregivers are often increasingly called on to make decisions. The increasing involvement of one individual as simultaneous caregiver, informant, and decision maker can pose particular complexities for clinicians.

First, the caregiver's role in identifying problems, providing history and corroborating patient reports can create tensions if clinicians are called upon to negotiate between conflicting points of view offered by patient and caregiver. For instance, patients with early-moderate Alzheimer's can experience paranoia, manifesting as a conviction that their spouse is having an affair. Certainly, stressors such as a personality change in a spouse and the responsibilities of caregiving can make a caregiver desirous of another supportive relationship. Clinicians may find themselves in the uncomfortable position of siding with one party against another. While caregivers will provide critical information, particularly regarding function at home, clinicians must continue to genuinely listen to what patients have to say for themselves.

Second, with increasing disability, caregivers can experience both physical and psychological exhaustion. Clinicians should be aware that the strain on caregivers may not only affect the care they provide for patients, but also the judgments caregivers make as surrogate decision makers. As the well-being of the caregiver is central to dementia care, clinicians must attend to caregiver as well as patient needs, and in essence may find themselves caring for two patients instead of one.

Conceptual foundations for decision making in cognitive impairment

Modern bioethics widely accepts that after a clinician explains treatment options, their risks and potential benefits, a patient has a right to refuse any treatment. This practice of obtaining informed consent (sometimes referred to as "valid" consent) promotes patient autonomy and self-determination. Three essential components are necessary to ensure informed consent: adequate disclosure of information, voluntariness of the choice, and the patient must be competent to make the decision. For patients with dementia and progressive cognitive decline, competence may be difficult to meet.

EVIDENCE AT A GLANCE

Essential elements of informed consent
There are three essential elements of informed consent.

1. Disclosure : physicians must convey adequate information to the patient
2. Voluntariness : the patient's consent must be obtained freely
3. Competency: the patient must be competent to consent or refuse

---

Capacity versus competence

Although competency and decision-making capacity are closely related, a meaningful distinction between them exists. Decision-making capacity describes a person's decisional abilities. Decision-making capacity should not be thought of as an "all or nothing" trait. Instead, persons possess a degree of decision-making capacity, and this capacity can change over time.

In contrast, competency describes whether a person has adequate decision-making capacity to make a *particular* decision. Thus, a patient may be competent to select a treatment but not competent to decide whether to enroll in a research protocol. Deciding whether a patient is competent also requires considering the particular *context* and *consequences* of the decision. For instance, a patient taking medication to treat hypercholesterolemia might believe it works by "purging the liver." This incorrect belief suggests impairment in the patient's decision-making capacity (since the patient lacks true understanding of the treatment's mechanism of action). However, this misunderstanding presents minimal potential negative consequences for the patient. If the patient understood the purpose, risks, and benefits of the medicine to their health, it would be reasonable for clinicians to conclude that this patient is competent to make this decision.

★ TIPS AND TRICKS

Evaluating decision-making capacity versus competence
Decision-making capacity describes a patient's decisional abilities. In contrast, competency describes whether a patient has adequate decision-making capacity to make a *particular* decision.

Assessing decision-making capacity

There are four widely accepted abilities that constitute decision-making capacity: expressing a choice, understanding, appreciation, and reasoning (Box 10.1). The first ability is the simplest; patients must be able to clearly communicate a choice (e.g. "I do not want a feeding tube"). This choice should be relatively stable over time and not impulsive; thus, when patients express widely fluctuating choices physicians should consider if anxiety is playing a large role.

The second ability – understanding – means patients should be able to grasp significant relevant information which has been presented to them. Practically, this can be assessed by asking patients to paraphrase important information. For instance, the clinician can ask the patient, "Tell me in your own words what I told you about the steps we take to insert a feeding tube." The goal is to verify that important facts have been successfully communicated.

Deciding what level of understanding is acceptable requires clinicians to exercise judgment. For instance, a patient's inability to recall whether a tube might be placed in the duodenum versus the jejunum is unlikely to be problematic. In contrast, a patient who is unable to understand that feeding tube placement involves a surgical procedure raises significant concerns about their understanding of a significant fact. Because memory and language are critical for understanding, patients for whom these domains are impaired, such as Alzheimer's patients, can have significant difficulty meeting this standard.

While assessing a patient's understanding is primarily concerned with the successful communication of facts, the third ability – the ability to appreciate – requires patients to demonstrate an awareness of how these facts are *personally* meaningful. In other words, the patient must not only grasp the facts (e.g. "feeding tubes are for people who cannot get enough food by mouth"), but recognize how these facts relate to their individual situation (e.g. "I cannot swallow and that is why my doctor has talked to me about having a feeding tube").

Finally, the fourth ability, reasoning, requires a patient to analyze information they have received. Patients ought to display some ability to work through possible consequences of various alternatives and to compare options. The goal of this standard is not to pass judgment on which choice the patient makes, but rather to evaluate the process by which a patient arrives at that decision. Thus, to assess consequential reasoning, one might ask, "How would having a feeding tube affect your daily life?" Similarly, one might assess comparative reasoning by asking, "Why do you prefer not to have a feeding tube placed instead of having this procedure done?" Because the ability to weigh various risks and rewards relies heavily on executive function, patients with significant impairment in executive function such as frontotemporal dementia can find it particularly difficult to reason.

Standardized tools for assessing capacity exist, such as the MacArthur network instruments to assess research or treatment consent capacity. These instruments allow a clinician to thoroughly assess all the relevant abilities for a given decision and then exercise clinical judgment as to whether the patient lacks capacity, a judgment that involves deciding how much impairment in which abilities will describe a patient who lacks capacity.

BOX 10.1 Assessing Decision-Making Capacity

The ability to make and communicate a choice

Ask the patient to indicate a choice

The ability to understand

Ask the patient to paraphrase back information that has been provided regarding the medical condition and treatment

The ability to appreciate

Ask the patient to articulate potential outcomes and consequences associated with treatment or no treatment

The patient should demonstrate awareness of how these facts are relevant to their particular situation

The ability to reason

Ask the patient to provide an explanation of the process or rationale for arriving at the decision

The patient should be able to demonstrate awareness of various options and at least some ability to compare between them

Source: Appelbaum PS. Clinical practice. Assessment of patients' competence to consent to treatment. *N Engl J Med* 2007; **357**(18): 1834–40.

Important considerations when clinicians suspect that patients lack capacity

Clinicians should not assume that cognitive impairment is the only cause of impaired decision-making capacity. Many processes other than dementia can also impair capacity, including major depression, anxiety, and delirium arising from a variety of medical illnesses. These conditions can be quite prevalent in older patients, particularly those with dementia. In fact, distinguishing whether symptoms stem from dementia or depression can be a challenging task, sometimes requiring dedicated neuropsychological testing. The prevalence of depression, a potentially treatable condition, in Alzheimer's patients has been estimated to be as high as 30%. Therefore, when clinicians suspect a loss of decision-making capacity, it is important consider all possible causes, not only dementia, particularly as some causes may be amenable to treatment and some degree of decision-making capacity can be restored.

✋ CAUTION

Depression can mimic cognitive dysfunction resulting from progressive dementia. As the prevalence of depression in Alzheimer's dementia can be as high as 30%, clinicians should always screen for depression in patients with decreased decision-making capacity.

Although measures of overall cognition, such as the Mini-Mental Status Examination (MMSE), correlate well with clinical judgments of incapacity and can provide a reasonable first step in gauging competence, cognition cannot substitute for a capacity assessment. While studies differ regarding the precise boundaries, broadly speaking, in patients with a MMSE >24, decision-making capacity is generally preserved. Conversely, patients with a MMSE <18 are likely to have significant impairments in decision-making capacity, especially as scores drop below 10.

EVIDENCE AT A GLANCE

Generally, patients with a MMSE >24 have preserved decision-making capacity. Conversely, patients with a MMSE <18 are likely to have significant impairments in decision-making capacity, especially as scores drop below 10.

Finally, it is important to recognize that even when patients possess full decision-making capacity, they have the right to cede the task of deciding to another, possibly a family member or caregiver, very possibly their physician. Clinicians should recognize a patient's wish to yield decision making to another as a fully valid expression of individual autonomy.

Surrogate decision making: substituted judgment or best interests

As decision-making capacity decreases, caregivers take on the additional role of surrogate decision maker. Two standards drawn from the law may offer guidance for caregivers in how to approach decisions: substituted judgment and best interests. Each reflects a distinct philosophy about how a surrogate decision maker should decide on behalf of a patient who cannot decide for themselves.

A substituted judgment standard argues that the decision maker should reconstruct what decision the patient would have made, if she found herself in that particular situation. Drawing on knowledge of the patient's beliefs, values and priorities, the surrogate should choose *as the patient would have chosen*. In contrast, the best interests standard suggests the surrogate decision maker should decide what is best for the patient, not attempt to surmise what she would theoretically have chosen.

EVIDENCE AT A GLANCE

Traditionally, two broad approaches exist to guide surrogate decision makers. According to the **substituted judgment** standard, drawing on knowledge of the patient's beliefs, values and priorities, the surrogate should choose *as the patient would have chosen* if she found herself in that particular situation. In contrast, according to the **best interests** standard, a surrogate decision maker should decide based on what is in the best interests of the patient, not what she would theoretically have chosen.

One way to distinguish these contrasting views is to describe the substituted judgment approach as primarily concerned with preserving patient autonomy (i.e. trying to decide what the patient would have decided) while the best interests approach prioritizes beneficence (choosing what the surrogate considers best for the patient, regardless of what she would have wanted).

Dementia's typically gradual course of decline means that patients have the opportunity to consider and express their future wishes with loved ones who may eventually serve as surrogate decision makers. Thus, some ethicists have argued that a surrogate ought to begin by first following any explicit wishes the patient may have expressed, followed by a substituted judgment approach when facing decisions where prior knowledge of patient beliefs allows extrapolation. Finally, when challenged with decisions for which they have no knowledge of what the patient might have valued, surrogates ought to adopt a best interests approach, choosing what they think is best for the patient.

While this tiered model provides useful structure, putting it into practice presents practical complexities. First, substituted judgments are often inaccurate. One study of patients and their designated surrogates demonstrated that surrogates using a substituted judgment framework to decide about future medical scenarios such as stroke or Alzheimer's were inaccurate >30% of the time. Furthermore, when inaccurate, surrogates consistently chose *more* aggressive care compared to what patients stated they would choose for themselves. Providing surrogates with a copy of an advance directive completed by the patient did not improve the accuracy of surrogate predictions.

EVIDENCE AT A GLANCE

Adopting a substituted judgment approach to surrogate decision making is challenging because surrogate decision makers are often inaccurate at predicting what a loved one would want. One study of patients and their designated surrogates demonstrated that surrogates using a substituted judgment framework to decide about future medical scenarios such as stroke or Alzheimer's were inaccurate >30% of the time.

These findings are consistent with the observations of many practitioners involved in end-of-life care. Even when patients leave explicit instructions to withdraw care, it is common for family members to intuitively feel guilty about "abandoning" a loved one when making these decisions. These discrepancies raise significant questions about whether a substituted judgment paradigm for surrogate decision making is realistic.

In defense of substituted judgment, one might argue that even if surrogates make inaccurate predictions, retaining patient wishes as the primary driving factor represents the best hope for decisions to approach what the patient would have wanted. However, this approach must balance at least three considerations.

First, surrogates are also often the primary caregiver and subject to stressors which may significantly affect decisions. For instance, depressed caregivers are less likely to choose cardiopulmonary resuscitation (CPR) for their loved ones. Second, while patients may discuss their treatment preferences with surrogates, for most patients, it is difficult to fully anticipate what they might want in a given situation. Thus, a patient might express a strong desire to "do everything." However, in practice, even this "ultimatum" may present significant ambiguities: should a surrogate enroll this patient in a trial that offers a 50:50 chance of significant improvement versus significant decline? Occasionally, patients with amyotrophic lateral sclerosis, another incurable neurodegenerative disease, will initially find it inconceivable to imagine consenting to a feeding tube, but change their mind when faced with the reality of swallowing dysfunction. The limited ability of patients to foresee and convey preferences for a multitude of potential scenarios, at a minimum severely limits the situations in which substituted judgment is useful. Third, it is not clear that patients themselves always want their wishes to be followed to the letter. In one study of patients receiving dialysis, two-thirds expressed the desire for their surrogates to exercise "leeway" when interpreting their advance directives should they develop Alzheimer's disease. Thus, even patients themselves express reservation about surrogates strictly adhering to their instructions in light of future uncertainties.

EVIDENCE AT A GLANCE

Evidence suggests patients themselves do not always want their wishes to be followed to the letter. In one study of patients receiving dialysis, two-thirds expressed the desire for their surrogates to exercise "leeway" when interpreting their advance directives should they develop Alzheimer's disease. Thus, even patients themselves express reservation about surrogates strictly adhering to their instructions given future uncertainties.

Substituted interests model

To address the challenges of implementing either one of these approaches in isolation, Sulmasy and Snyder have proposed a blended "substituted interests model" as an alternative. This model acknowledges that attempts to preserve patient autonomy by divining what a patient would have decided in a given situation are ultimately futile and highly stressful for surrogates. Instead, surrogates are asked to speak in their capacity as experts regarding the patient's values and beliefs. A surrogate's testimony to distinctive values which characterize a patient provides the foundation for a constructive conversation between clinician and surrogate about what the real interests of the patient might be. Drawing on this knowledge, clinicians can offer surrogates information and guidance on ways in which this patient's unique profile of interests might be honored in the particular clinical context. Together, clinicians and surrogates can then participate in the process of shared decision making, judging what course of medical action most authentically represent the patient's interests.

The substituted interests model differs from its predecessors in two distinctive ways. First, according to the substituted judgment and best interests standards, decision-making responsibility rests solely on the surrogate's shoulders. In contrast, the substituted interests model acknowledges that the heavy responsibility of decision making should be shared between clinicians and surrogates (although ultimate decision continues to rest with the surrogate). Second, where uncertainty exists regarding what the patient would have wanted, decisions are driven by knowledge of the patient's core values and beliefs, instead of attempts to guess the details of what specific decision the patient would have made. For example, a substituted judgment standard asks the surrogate to determine what particular *judgment* (i.e. decision) the patient would have made (i.e. "I am sure my father would never have chosen a feeding tube"). Instead, the substituted interests model proposes that the surrogate and physician's task is to determine what decision best represents the patient's known *interests*, i.e. "Two things my father deeply valued were spirited conversations with family and living without pain. Alzheimer's has made such conversations no longer possible and he has developed painful bedsores and trouble swallowing. Although he never specifically discussed feeding tube placement,

having a feeding tube placed to keep him alive would not be in keeping with the things he valued – like relating to family and living pain free."

Importantly, in this model, specific instructions which the patient left should certainly continue to guide decisions. However, this model suggests that patients should be encouraged to discuss not only specific medical decisions but how strictly instructions should be followed. This substituted interests approach preserves the commitment to patient-centeredness which motivates substituted judgment, but acknowledges that particularly where ambiguity exists, surrogates and clinicians can use the patient's values to infer what decision best reflects the patient's interests.

EVIDENCE AT A GLANCE

The substituted interests model combines elements of the substituted judgment and best interests standards for surrogate decision making. According to the substituted interests model, the surrogate provides information on the patient's distinctive values. The physician then informs the surrogate of ways in which those values might be enacted given the particular medical context. Together, physician and surrogate discuss what decision best represents the patient's known *interests*. While this is a process of shared decision making, the ultimate decision-making power continues to rest with the surrogate.

In practice, surrogate decision makers often employ a process resembling a substituted interests approach, combining various elements of the substituted judgment and best interests approaches, particularly once patients have progressed to advanced dementia. Hirschman and colleagues found that few surrogates adopted the use of a substituted judgment standard alone; instead, most endorsed either a best interests approach or some combination of the two. Similarly, a survey of terminally ill patients, performed by Sulmasy and colleagues, found that most patients prefer for surrogates to use a mixture of the substituted judgment and best interests approaches when making decisions. Thus, clinicians should reassure surrogates that they should not only consider any preferences their loved one may have expressed, but also what they see as providing the most benefit and quality of life to their loved one. For instance, clinicians might offer caregivers guidance with a statement such as: "Two useful guides as you think about what we should do are to think about what your husband would have wanted if he could tell us what to do and what will maximize his dignity and quality of life."

★ TIPS AND TRICKS

Clinicians should reassure surrogates that they should not only consider any preferences their loved one may have expressed, but also what they see as providing the most benefit and quality of life to their loved one. For instance, clinicians might offer caregivers guidance with a statement such as: "Two useful guides as you think about what we should do are to think about what your husband would have wanted if he could tell us what to do and what will maximize his dignity and quality of life."

Common issues for clinicians

Clinicians who care for patients with dementia will face common issues, including participation in research, advance directives, driving, voting, screening for elder abuse, and caring for caregivers.

Participation in research

Because existing treatments for Alzheimer's disease and other common causes of dementia offer only limited efficacy, patients often ask about enrolling in research, particularly research involving development of new treatments. However, dementia patients constitute an inherently vulnerable research population; once decision-making capacity is impaired, someone other than the patient will be tasked with deciding on the patient's behalf.

Deciding whether participation in clinical research is appropriate involves weighing possible benefits against potential harms. This balancing is ethically complex if research offers potential for substantial value to the general public, but is unlikely to directly benefit an individual patient. Several professional society guidelines have emphasized the importance of prioritizing direct benefit to the patient when considering whether recruitment among cognitively impaired patients should be allowed. Given the history of prior abuse to vulnerable populations, these protective measures are understandable. However, there may be unintended consequences. For instance, excluding these patients from all trials without potential direct benefit could paradoxically expose them to higher risk from non-dementia related drugs which have never been tested in this population before coming to market. Also, by sharply limiting patient participation when no direct benefit is likely, these ethical guidelines express a viewpoint which prioritizes concern for the individual. However, a noteworthy number of patients facing life-threatening disease find it deeply meaningful for altruistic reasons to participate in research to benefit future patients, fully knowing that they themselves are unlikely to benefit. The perspective of these patients raises important questions regarding whether the current paradigm has emphasized protecting the individual in ways which ironically limit the ability of current patients to contribute towards the well-being of future patients.

Currently, consensus exists that non-competent subjects should be allowed to participate in research that meets either of the following criteria: research must (1) present some reasonable prospect of benefit to the subjects or (2) if it does not present such a prospect, the research must present only minimal risk and potentially yield important information for a class of subjects addressed by the study. When research presents no benefit and more than minimal risk, some guidelines have required that the potential participant should have previously expressed a wish to participate in such research. Finally, the subject must be able to assent, a standard drawn from pediatric research, in which subjects are acknowledged to be unable to provide full informed consent, but capable of expressing either willingness or unwillingness (i.e. "assent" or "dissent") to participate in research when provided with basic information.

Regarding the question of who will provide consent, federal law stipulates that for adults, a third party (a "legalized authorized representative" or LAR, often referred to as a proxy or surrogate) may provide consent for participation in research. However, criteria defining LAR, or whether additional protections should apply for consent obtained from surrogates, were left for states to decide and for most part, remain unclear. There is certainly evidence of public support for the validity of surrogate consent in this context. Scott Kim and colleagues surveyed adults at risk for Alzheimer's and found strong support for surrogates to consent even when studies offered no direct benefit, particularly when the risks of research were low. Notably, a majority continued to find consent by a surrogate on their behalf acceptable, even for research scenarios that involved significant risks, such as a brain biopsy.

> **EVIDENCE AT A GLANCE**
>
> Should surrogates be able to enroll patients in research studies? A survey of adults at risk for Alzheimer's found strong support for surrogates to consent even when studies offered no direct benefit, particularly when the risks of research were low. A majority continued to find consent by a surrogate on their behalf acceptable, even for research scenarios that involved significant risks, such as a brain biopsy.

In some cases, surrogates may decline to give consent for patient participation in research, despite some indications (e.g. patient assent) suggesting the patient may be inclined to participate. As robust clinical trial enrollment remains a key challenge to moving research forward, some have sought to address this issue by encouraging advance directives which state a patient's desire for future participation in research. However, adoption of this type of advance directive has been extremely low, and there is some evidence that patient willingness to cede the decision about trial enrollment to a surrogate in the future may vary depending on the type of research.

Finally, clinician-investigators should remain mindful that although patients may become unable to consent for themselves, they may still possess sufficient decisional capability to meaningfully contribute to the decision-making process. Stocking and colleagues found that dementia patients were generally comfortable with ceding decision making to a proxy; however, their comfort with allowing surrogates to decide decreased as the potential risks of various research scenarios increased. In fact, one-third of patients expressed concern for allowing a surrogate to decide in at least one out of five research scenarios presented. This may suggest that even at

late stages of disease, dementia patients retain some ability to differentiate levels of risk or designate a proxy decision maker.

> **EVIDENCE AT A GLANCE**
>
> Even in advanced stages of dementia, patients may be able to meaningfully contribute to decisions. One survey found that dementia patients were increasingly reluctant to cede decision making about research enrollment to a surrogate with increasing potential risks of various research scenarios.

Advance directives

In addition to delegating decision-making power to another individual by designating a surrogate decision maker, healthcare proxy or Durable Power Of Attorney, patients can also describe their wishes by writing an advance directive. The 1990 Patient Self Determination Act mandated that all facilities receiving Medicare/Medicaid funds were required to inform patients of the right to record their wishes using an advance directive. This legislation was intended to increase awareness and adoption. However, although advance directives were once widely regarded as the key to ensuring that patient preferences for care (particularly at the end of life) would be met, challenges arising from limited usage and implementation of these directives are now generally acknowledged by long-time advocates for improving end-of-life care. Certainly, the care most patients receive at the end of life presents opportunities for advance directives to be useful. Silveira and colleagues found that 70% of patients requiring medical decision making in the final days of life lacked decision-making capacity and, not surprisingly, patients with cognitive impairment were at significantly increased risk of lacking capacity. Of these patients for whom a decision was required, 30% lacked an advance directive. Furthermore, even when patients have clearly written directives, the degree to which these documents significantly influence the use of life support remains unclear.

Three factors in particular may limit the usefulness of advance directives. First, the language of these documents often specifies a patient's wishes in the event that they are faced with the prospect of no meaningful recovery. However, prognostic uncertainty and a lack of clarity regarding what constitutes "meaningful" often render the advance directive unhelpful. Second, even when patient wishes are clearly stated (i.e. "I do not want to have a feeding tube placed"), strong opposition by family members can make physicians reluctant to implement the patient's wishes. Third, while decisions may be informed by an advance directive, decisions are often ultimately made by a surrogate, often a family member. Despite explicit instructions to continue life support, surrogates may find it difficult to comply if they feel their loved one is suffering; conversely, it may be difficult to withdraw care, if surrogates feel that they are "giving up" on their loved one.

Although advance directives remain a flawed tool, the process of considering one's wishes, writing an advanced directive, and discussing preferences with family members is undoubtedly helpful. Dementia patients will almost certainly lack capacity to make end-of-life decisions and physicians should encourage patients to consider writing an advance directive. Undoubtedly, the timing of these discussions requires sensitivity; raising this topic at diagnosis is almost never necessary in dementia given the typical pace of disease progression and only creates additional stress for patients and families at an already difficult moment. However, clinicians should begin these conversations relatively early to ensure that patients are able to contemplate and convey personal preferences to their families before cognitive impairment makes this difficult or impossible. To introduce this during a clinic visit, a clinician can ask the patient, "It's important for you to communicate your wishes for care with your loved ones to help them make better decisions on your behalf in the future. Have you given this some thought?" Given the potential barriers discussed above, clinicians should emphasize that patients should discuss the contents of their advance directive with surrogate decision makers and other family members.

> ☆ **TIPS AND TRICKS**
>
> To introduce the topic of advanced directives during a clinic visit, a clinician might suggest, "It's important for you to communicate your wishes for care with your loved ones to help them make better decisions on your behalf in the future. Have you given this some thought?"

Although advance directives are legally binding, preparing one does not require a lawyer, making the process relatively inexpensive, with the only costs being those associated with using a public notary. Advance directives are valid in all 50 states, but laws governing language and use differ from state to state. Patients and families can use the National Hospice and Palliative Care Organization webpage that describes advance directives and provides templates which meet specific standards for each particular state (www.caringinfo.org/i4a/pages/index.cfm?pageid=3287).

> ☆ **TIPS AND TRICKS**
>
> Patients and families can be directed to the National Hospice and Palliative Care Organization webpage which describes advance directives and provides templates meeting state-specific standards (www.caringinfo.org/i4a/pages/index.cfm?pageid=3287).

Driving

The topic of driving restrictions may be among the most difficult conversations clinicians face in caring for patients with dementia. For many patients, the ability to drive is synonymous with independence and thus deeply tied to a sense of self. Losing the ability to drive can be a symbolic moment for both patients and caregivers, bringing not only new pragmatic challenges but grief at a sense of lost liberty. Without the ability to drive, many patients may find participation in social activities more difficult, becoming increasingly isolated and at greater risk for depression.

As driving is central to many aspects of life, patients may naturally become angry or feel betrayed when this issue is raised, particularly if they lack insight into their deficits. In the face of fierce opposition, clinicians may find it difficult to take away such a cherished activity. However, driving is a privilege, not a right. Furthermore, clinicians are charged with not only the well-being of the patient, but guarding public safety. In fact, in some states, physicians are mandated to report when patients are no longer safe to drive, and in some cases, there may be repercussions for physicians who do not comply.

As the potential for harm to patients and others is so significant, clinicians should be alert for signs of impaired driving ability. Accidents and citations for reckless driving are obvious signs, but aggressive or impulsive behavior should also trigger caution. While the MMSE is not a good predictor of driving performance, the Clinical Disease Rating (CDR) scale has been demonstrated to correlate well with degree of driving impairment. Patients with a CDR of 0.5 are mildly impaired and should be encouraged to avoid driving or limit their driving to particular hours (i.e. daytime) or shorter distances. A CDR of 1 suggests the patient poses a significant traffic safety risk and should be strongly advised not to drive. Clinically, patients with a CDR of 1 will have memory impairment interfering with everyday activities; also, these patients will have given up complicated activities or hobbies and require prompting to maintain personal grooming. A complete description of the CDR can be found at http://rgp.toronto.on.ca/dmcourse/toolkit/app5.htm.

EVIDENCE AT A GLANCE

The Clinical Disease Rating (CDR) scale correlates well with degree of driving impairment. Patients with a CDR of 0.5 are mildly impaired and should be encouraged to avoid driving or limit their driving to particular hours (i.e. daytime). A CDR of 1 suggests that the patient poses a significant traffic safety risk and should be strongly advised not to drive.

Strategies that may decrease the chances of confrontation over driving include early and open conversations about how dementia affects driving skills. These conversations can prepare patients for future restrictions and provide occasion for caregivers to share any concerns they may have about their loved one driving. Second, referral for a driving evaluation (available at many rehabilitation facilities) may persuade some patients of the extent to which their deficits have progressed. Occupational therapists can also provide judgments about a patient's ability to drive safely. For caregivers and patients, driving may prove a point of contention, with caregivers becoming increasingly reluctant to allow the patient to drive as other deficits develop. Where uncertainty remains, one useful rule of thumb is to ask the patient's family if they would feel comfortable having their grandchildren or someone else's grandchildren driven around by the patient. Unless the answer is clearly "yes," further assessment of the patient's driving ability should be pursued.

Voting

Older citizens make up a significant proportion of voters, but also the segment of the population with the highest prevalence of dementia. Given the progressive nature of dementia, every year a number of older citizens previously capable of voting will lose this ability due to cognitive impairment. Conversely, many elderly individuals may retain the cognitive capacities needed to vote, but are impeded by logistical barriers (i.e. limited mobility, no clear nursing home policy). The potential for influence or abuse of voting privileges by caregivers who may be instrumental in obtaining and marking absentee ballots (i.e. voting fraud) adds a further layer of complexity.

Although the question of voting may not commonly arise during a doctor's visit, it is important for clinicians to be aware of the issues and become educated advocates for clarity and improved access for cognitively impaired patients cared for at home and in nursing facilities. Efforts include facilitating registration and absentee ballot use, and, for nursing home residents, mobile polling, a process whereby election officials go to a long-term care facility and assist residents who want to vote.

Elder abuse

In 2009, it was estimated that there were 2 million cases of elder self-neglect or abuse in the United States, with an increasing yearly number of reported cases. Elder abuse can take many forms, but refers to any knowing, intentional or negligent acts by a caregiver or any other person that causes serious risk of harm to a vulnerable adult. The National Center on Elder Abuse (NCEA) identifies three broad categories of abuse: abuse by caregivers, institutions (such as nursing facilities), and self-neglect. The harm inflicted may be physical or sexual, but may also take the form of emotional violence or financial exploitation. Patients with memory problems are known to be at increased risk for abuse. Similarly, particular characteristics may place caregivers at higher risk for becoming abusers. An estimated two-thirds of abusers are family members, typically spouses or children. Specifically, caregivers who feel overwhelmed or resentful, have a history of substance abuse or physical abuse of others, or are dependent on the patient for financial support or housing needs may be at increased risk for becoming abusive.

✋ CAUTION

Roughly two-thirds of abusers are family members, typically spouses or children. Caregivers who feel overwhelmed or resentful, have a history of substance abuse or physical abuse of others, or are dependent on the patient for financial support or housing needs may be at increased risk for becoming abusive.

Not only is elder abuse distressing on moral and ethical grounds, it may be associated with increased risk of death. Dong and colleagues demonstrated that self-neglect and elder abuse are associated with increased risk of mortality; notably, this increased mortality risk was not restricted to patients with more severe cognitive or physical impairments. Clinicians should be alert for signs of abuse or neglect such as patient withdrawal from usual activities, sudden changes in personality or behavior, unexplained bruises or angry exchanges between caregiver and patient. The NCEA offers significant resources, including materials for caregivers under pressure who may worry about becoming abusive. In addition, clinicians can report abuse and locate local state services by using the elder care helpline (1-800-677-1116).

★ TIPS AND TRICKS

Signs of patient abuse or neglect include patient withdrawal from usual activities, sudden changes in personality or behavior, unexplained bruises or angry exchanges between caregiver and patient. Report abuse and locate local state services by using the elder care helpline (1-800-677-1116).

Recent cases, such as that involving Stephanie Hernandez, highlight the complexities of assigning blame. Hernandez, who had cared for her 91-year-old great-aunt Concha Lopez for 3 years, was charged with elder abuse and murder after it was discovered that Lopez had died at home with multiple bed sores, covered with feces, and weighing a scant 35 lbs. However, before becoming bedbound and developing severe dementia, Lopez had expressed a strong aversion to doctors and begged her family to spare her from dying in a hospital facility. Hernandez was incarcerated for over a year before being acquitted of all charges, but the case illustrates how difficult it can be for caregivers, particularly those with limited resources, to honor the wishes of loved ones with dementia. As the number of cognitively impaired adults cared for at home continues to increase, the challenges of ensuring that caregivers provide appropriate care that honors patient preferences will only increase.

Caring for caregivers

The majority of adults requiring long-term care currently live at home cared for by unpaid caregivers. Specifically, unpaid family caregivers provide care for 80% of Alzheimer's disease patients who remain at home. Providing care for cognitively impaired patients can prove particularly demanding since patients typically require higher levels of supervision compared to patients with other chronic illnesses. In addition, roughly one-quarter of caregivers also have children under 18 and nearly half (44%) continue to work full or part time. This caretaking can exact a toll with up to 80% of Alzheimer's disease caregivers reporting high levels of stress and half reporting depression. Patients with aggressive or agitated behaviors or nighttime wandering can prove particularly challenging to care for, especially if caregivers cannot obtain adequate rest. In more severe stages of disease, it is not uncommon for caregivers to report feeling as if they are "on duty 24 hours a day."

Identifying signs of caregiver stress and burnout is an important part of the clinician's task in dementia. Well-established tools for screening for caregiver burden exist, such as the Zarit Caregiver Burden Scale and the Caregiver Strain Index (CSI). One fast and easily administered screening tool, developed for clinic use by Hirschmann and colleagues, is composed of seven questions derived from the 25-item Screen for Caregiver Burden. This covers various common domains of potential stress which can be recalled using the pneumonic ABCD-RIK, which stands for: Alone, Behaviors, Chores, Difficulty communicating,

Repetitive questions, Illness and Keeping the House in order (Box 10.2). The tool's simplicity allows it to be administered by a medical assistant or completed by the caregiver while the patient's vital signs are being taken, thus providing this information to clinicians without requiring additional time during the visit.

Depending on the source of stress, caregivers may benefit from referral to social service agencies to identify greater home services or arrange for respite care. A variety of interventions including support groups and educational interventions have improved caregiver skill, knowledge, and well-being as well as depressive symptoms and in some cases, delayed time to nursing home placement. Patient advocacy organizations, such as the Alzheimer's Association, maintain helpful resources for caregivers to monitor their own stress levels and suggestions for managing the daily stressors of patient care (www.alz.org/living_with_alzheimers_caring_for_alzheimers.asp).

Broader social and cultural reflections

In addition to the issues already discussed, distinctive features of American culture present additional ethical challenges to dementia patients and their families. In general, images of the young, sharp, and healthy have claimed cultural precedence. Because the ability to choose or decide for oneself is highly prized in modern society and considered foundational to so many aspects of life, perhaps it is not surprising that conversely, aging is increasingly understood primarily in terms of various deficiencies. This emphasis on youth, vigor, and capacity is ethically concerning as it suggests a devaluation of older persons, especially those with physical and cognitive limitations. The relative sequestration of the elderly out of public view, either in nursing homes or in the homes of family caregivers, adds to this concern. This tendency to keep impaired persons relatively hidden may suggest that despite advances made towards understanding the biology of common causes of dementia, there is still something shameful about Alzheimer's disease. In addition to working towards identifying further causes and treatments for dementia, it is also important for clinicians and researchers to remain aware of these cultural dynamics and work to affirm the dignity and value of patients with dementia, despite their cognitive limitations.

Providing care for patients with dementia and their families presents complex legal, ethical, and social issues. Much of the clinician's task focuses on addressing practical challenges that will confront patients and families and, where possible, offering guidance and practical support. The issues addressed in this chapter can be among the most difficult to negotiate for patients and families. When President Ronald Reagan was diagnosed with Alzheimer's disease, he wrote the American public: "I now begin the journey that will lead me into the sunset of my life." Although every patient's path will be unique, a thoughtful appreciation of the ethical, legal, and social issues at stake in dementia will make clinicians better partners as they take this journey with patients and families.

Box 10.2 Seven-item screen for caregiver burden. Caregivers are asked to rate whether each of the following experiences or events occurred and caused them stress, or did not occur	
Alone	1. I feel so alone – as if I have the world on my shoulders.
Behavior	2. I have little control over my relative's behavior.
Chores	3. I have to do too many jobs/chores (feeding, shopping) that my relative used to do.
Difficulty communicating	4. I am upset that I cannot communicate with my relative.
Repetitive questions	5. My relative is constantly asking the same questions over and over.
Illness	6. I have little control over my relative's illness.
Keeping the house in order	7. My relative does not cooperate with the rest of our family.

Reproduced from Kirschman K, et al. The development of a rapid screen for caregiver burden. *J Am Geriatr Soc* 2004; **52**: 1724–9, with permission from Wiley.

Further reading

Appelbaum PS. Clinical practice. Assessment of patients' competence to consent to treatment. *N Engl J Med* 2007; **357**(18): 1834–40.

Ditto PH, Danks JH, Smucker WD, et al. Advance directives as acts of communication: a randomized controlled trial. *Arch Intern Med* 2001; **161**(3): 421–30.

Dong X, Simon M, Mendes de Leon C, et al. Elder self-neglect and abuse and mortality risk in a community-dwelling population. *JAMA* 2009; **302**(5): 517–26.

Hirschman KB, Shea JA, Xie SX, Karlawish JH. The development of a rapid screen for caregiver burden. *J Am Geriatr Soc* 2004; **52**(10): 1724–9.

Karlawish JH, Bonnie RJ, Appelbaum PS, et al. Addressing the ethical, legal, and social issues raised by voting by persons with dementia. *JAMA* 2004; **292**(11): 1345–50.

Karlawish JH, Casarett D, Klocinski J, Sankar P. How do AD patients and their caregivers decide whether to enroll in a clinical trial? *Neurology* 2001; **56**(6): 789–92.

Kim SY, Kim HM, McCallum C, Tariot PN. What do people at risk for Alzheimer disease think about surrogate consent for research? *Neurology* 2005; **65**(9): 1395–401.

Lo B. Assessing decision-making capacity. *Law Med Health Care* 1990; **18**(3): 193–201.

Muthappan P, Forster H, Wendler D. Research advance directives: protection or obstacle? *Am J Psychiatry* 2005; **162**(12): 2389–91.

Sehgal A, Galbraith A, Chesney M, Schoenfeld P, Charles G, Lo B. How strictly do dialysis patients want their advance directives followed? *JAMA* 1992; **267**(1): 59–63.

Silveira MJ, Kim SY, Langa KM. Advance directives and outcomes of surrogate decision making before death. *N Engl J Med*; **362**(13): 1211–18.

Stocking CB, Hougham GW, Danner DD, Patterson MB, Whitehouse PJ, Sachs GA. Speaking of research advance directives: planning for future research participation. *Neurology* 2006; **66**(9): 1361–6.

Sulmasy DP, Snyder L. Substituted interests and best judgments: an integrated model of surrogate decision making. *JAMA*; **304**(17): 1946–7.

Sulmasy DP, Hughes MT, Thompson RE, et al. How would terminally ill patients have others make decisions for them in the event of decisional incapacity? A longitudinal study. *J Am Geriatr Soc* 2007; **55**(12): 1981–8.

White DB, Arnold RM. The evolution of advance directives. *JAMA* 2011; **306**(13): 1485–6.

11

Assessing Outcomes in Dementia Care

Joel Mack,[1] Amie Peterson[2] and Joseph Quinn[2]

[1] Department of Psychiatry, Oregon Health and Science University, USA
[2] Department of Neurology, Oregon Health and Science University, USA

Introduction

In his thought-provoking book *Better*, Atul Gawande points out two examples of advances in medicine which relied on quantification of outcomes. The first example is obstetrics, where the introduction of the simple Apgar scoring system for neonatal health permitted comparison of outcomes between different obstetric methods and ultimately led to dramatic declines in neonatal morbidity and mortality. The second example is the treatment of cystic fibrosis, which is based on pulmonary function goals. By applying simple algorithms for optimizing pulmonary function, in the absence of any real scientific advances, cystic fibrosis clinics have increased the average lifespan of cystic fibrosis patients from less than 6 years to greater than 40 years. These stories illustrate the power of careful definition of therapeutic goals and outcome measures. If dramatic improvements are possible in cystic fibrosis, surely some improved outcomes are possible in dementia care.

Comprehensive dementia care involves considering outcomes across a number of domains. While cognitive decline is the core problem in dementia, difficulties related to day-to-day function and quality of life, neuropsychiatric symptoms, caregiver distress, co-morbid medical issues, nursing home placement, and ultimately mortality are important to consider in the multidimensional approach required to treat dementia. However, cognitive impairment and these related problems do not allow for simple external observation, as most dementia symptoms are not of the type

detected on a physical neurological exam. How then should we develop the equivalent of an "Apgar score" for dementia care? The first step lies in utilizing valid and reliable measures that capture progression of the disease across various domains. Outcome measures for the clinical setting should also be convenient to use, adequately sensitive to change (with the goal of revealing disease progression over annual intervals), and useful across dementia stages.

Development and utilization of valid rating scales are essential for this reason, and there are currently a number of clinician-, caregiver-, and patient-rated instruments available that can be incorporated into clinical practice to track outcomes in dementia care. Assessing some outcomes, such as mortality, may be difficult because they are less frequent and may be affected by a number of other factors. Despite potential difficulties, improving our ability to track clinical dementia outcomes in quantifiable way, as has been done in other areas of medicine, will allow us to assess and compare dementia care across institutions, encourage the development of best practice, and ultimately improve the overall quality of care for dementia patients.

There is another practical reason to attempt to define ideal outcomes in dementia care. Reimbursement rates are likely to depend on achieving outcome goals in the not too distant future. The large variations in rates of healthcare utilization and clinical outcomes across geographic areas and institutions observed over the last 20 years have led to a shift from the traditional approach of relying on the

Dementia, First Edition. Edited by Joseph F. Quinn.
© 2014 John Wiley & Sons, Ltd. Published 2014 by John Wiley & Sons, Ltd.

medical profession to self-regulate delivery of uniform, quality healthcare. As a result, insurance companies, including Medicare, and governing bodies are implementing programs based on pay for performance, in which healthcare providers are rewarded for meeting predetermined healthcare delivery quality targets (or penalized for shortfalls). Such quality measures may be based on *structure* (inputs into the healthcare production process, e.g. whether a dementia patient is treated by their primary care doctor or a dementia specialist), *process* (procedures of diagnosis and treatment, e.g. whether or not a dementia patient had neuroimaging as part of their work-up), or *outcomes* (the end result of medical care, e.g. morbidity, mortality, quality of life, etc.). Ultimately, better outcomes are the goal of quality improvement measures and what patients and clinicians consider most important. The design and implementation of pay for performance programs as related to reimbursement are a complex endeavor at the systems level that must consider factors such as quality, cost, and access to care. As clinicians, taking the lead to improve outcomes in our day-to-day care of dementia patients will inform what performance measures are incorporated into pay for performance programs and allow us to make our voices heard as these programs become a reality.

Promoting evidence-based standardization of practices and outcomes measures is the first step in improving the quality of dementia care. In the United States, the National Institute of Aging (NIA) has designated 29 Alzheimer's disease centers (ADC), with the goal of establishing a dementia research network, but also to offer diagnosis, management, education, and support services to dementia patients and their families. Implemented in 2005, the NIA-ADC Uniform Data Set (UDS; see Tips and Tricks) is a standardized battery of measurements administered longitudinally at ADCs to track cognitive and functional decline in impaired individuals and the onset of cognitive change in those who were non-demented at initial assessment.

Domain assessed	Assessment instrument
Cognition	
General cognitive	Mini-Mental State Examination
verbal recall	Wechsler Memory Scale-Revised Logical memory IA immediate
Delayed verbal recall	Wechsler Memory Scale-Revised Logical memory IA delayed
Attention	Digit span forward and backward
Executive function	Trailmaking test-part B
Psychomotor speed	Trailmaking test-part A Wechsler Adult Intelligence Scale, revised digit symbol
Language	Category fluency (animals, vegetable) Boston Naming Test
Functional status	Functional Assessment Questionnaire
Behavioral assessment	Neuropsychiatric Inventory-Questionnaire Geriatric Depression Scale

While the development of the UDS was mainly research driven, its goal of providing a common set of clinical observations to be collected over time serves as an established standard for discussing outcomes in dementia care at the clinical level. While the UDS does not provide for comprehensive evaluation across the full range of domains, building on this model to develop a clinically relevant set of outcome measures for use in day to day practice will encourage quality improvement in dementia care. This chapter aims to describe some of the most commonly used, validated tools that may be used for tracking dementia outcomes across domains in the clinical setting, and to further highlight the role tracking outcomes may play in dementia care in the future.

★ TIPS AND TRICKS

Build on elements from the Uniform Data Set recommendations for neuropsychological, functional, and behavioral assessment to assess dementia outcomes

Cognition

Cognitive decline is the archetypal feature of all neurodegenerative dementias and is the source of other dementia-related problems. A full cognitive assessment, as part of the mental status examination, is the central element of a dementia work-up and subsequent follow-up over time. Initial assessment across cognitive areas, including memory, executive function, language, visuospatial skills, and praxis, is useful for differential consideration of dementia diagnosis and to understand a patient's particular cognitive strengths and weaknesses. Following diagnosis, degree of cognitive impairment provides an indicator of disease progression and response to interventions. There are a number of standardized cognitive examinations that aid in quantifying cognitive impairment. Many of these brief cognitive assessments were initially developed as screening tools for dementia or mild cognitive impairment (MCI) and not necessarily as rating scales (i.e. outcome measures) to assess progression of cognitive decline. Some scales may not be adequate or comparable for assessing non-Alzheimer's dementias. However, their reliability, convenience, and ability to provide a composite score that can be followed over time have led to their widespread use as outcome indicators in clinical settings.

Mini-Mental State Examination

The MMSE was originally designed to provide a brief, standardized assessment of mental status that would differentiate between organic and functional disorders in inpatient psychiatric patients, but has since become the most widely used brief cognitive assessment in dementia care. It is a 30-point scale assessing orientation (10 points), registration (3 points), attention and calculation (5 points), recall (3 points), and language (9 points). Administration time is typically about 10 min. In patients with dementia of the Alzheimer's type (AD), scores typically decline by 2–3 points per year, whereas frontotemporal dementia (FTD) patients decline at a rate as high as 6–7 points per year.

⚙ SCIENCE REVISITED

Annual rate of change scores for selected scales

- Mini-Mental State Exam (total score = 30)
  2–3 point decline in AD
  6–7 point decline in FTD

- Montreal Cognitive Assessment (total score = 30)
  2–3 point decline in AD
- Alzheimer's Disease Assessment Scale-Cognitive subscale (total score = 70)
  4–6 point increase in AD, with slower decline in early and late stages
- Neuropsychiatric Inventory (total score = 144)
  2–3 point increase in AD
- Clinical Dementia Rating Scale-Sum of Boxes score (total score = 18)
  1–2 point increase in AD

The widespread use of the MMSE over many years has the advantage of allowing comparisons across institutions or with historical patient records. The MMSE has been translated into a number of languages. Limitations include ceiling and floor effects, in which patients with high premorbid intelligence or education may not display impairment and patients with severe cognitive impairment score at the bottom of the range despite worsening dementia, respectively. Education-adjusted norms should be used for this reason. It is not particularly sensitive to MCI and also has limited use in assessing frontal-subcortical cognitive deficits. Additional testing may be needed to assess these areas.

Of note, the MMSE was copyrighted in 2001 and the official version must be ordered and paid for through Psychological Assessment Resources, Inc, which may make the test too costly for some settings.

Montreal Cognitive Assessment (MoCA)

The MoCA is a brief screening tool originally designed for detection of MCI. The total possible score is 30 points. It assesses various cognitive domains: attention and concentration (6 points), executive functions and conceptual thinking (4 points), memory (5 points), language (5 points), visuoconstructional skills (4 points), and orientation (6 points). Administration time is approximately 10 min. A score of 26 or above is considered normal. The rate of change in AD has been shown to be comparable to the MMSE. The MoCA's strength lies in its high sensitivity for both MCI and AD (90% and 100%, respectively). This makes it useful for screening and following patients with mild cognitive complaints who are not yet experiencing significant functional decline. In fact, due to some overlap in scores for MCI and AD, the suggested MoCA cut-off score is the same for both (<26), with the difference being accompanying functional decline in the case of AD. The MoCA can also be used in cases where cognitive impairment is suspected but the patient performs normally (>25) on the MMSE. The MoCA is available free at www.mocatest.org and has been translated into over 30 languages.

St Louis University Mental Status Examination (SLUMS)

Like the MoCA, the SLUMS was developed to be a more sensitive tool than the MMSE for detecting MCI. The SLUMS consists of 11 items, and measures aspects of cognition that include orientation (3 points), short-term memory (13 points), calculations (3 points), verbal fluency (3 points), working memory (2 points), and visuospatial ability (6 points, includes a clock draw). Scores range from 0 to 30, with scores of 27–30 considered normal in a person with a high school education. Scores between 21 and 26 suggest MCI, and scores between 0 and 20 indicate dementia. Administration time is typically about 7 min. Strengths of the SLUMS include the sensitivity to MCI, increased assessment of executive and visuospatial abilities compared to MMSE, and the use of two recall tasks, a five-word recall and a story recall. However, it is not as widely used as the MMSE and psychometric properties have not been as thoroughly validated. It is available free through the St Louis University medical school website.

> ### ✋ CAUTION
>
> Currently available instruments for assessing dementia outcomes may not be useful at all stages of dementia or across various dementia types. As examples, the MMSE may not be particularly sensitive to deficits in early dementia or frontal-subcortical dementias and the UDS recommendations were motivated by research priorities for MCI and AD, specifically. Future work should focus on developing better scales that capture outcomes across domains for specific dementia types and stages. In the meantime, clinical judgment is required to ensure that different or additional outcome measures are selected as necessary for comprehensive assessment of the various dementing illnesses.

Alzheimer's Disease Assessment Scale-Cognitive subscale (ADAS-Cog)

The ADAS-Cog should be mentioned as it is the cognitive outcome measure most widely used in trials of antidementia medications. It consists of 11 subtests examining memory, language, and praxis but lacks adequate testing of attention and executive function. Total scores range from 0 to 70, with higher scores (≥18) indicating greater cognitive impairment. A four-point change on the ADAS-Cog at 6 months has been recognized as indicating a clinically important difference in cognitive performance in clinical trials. However, the measurement error of the instrument has been thought by some to limit its use for assessing disease progression over the short term. Furthermore, the administration time for the ADAS-Cog typically is typically 30–45 min, depending on the stage of the patient's dementia, which may limit utility in the clinical setting.

Neuropsychological testing

Neuropsychological testing, as performed by a neuropsychologist, is an important tool employed in the diagnosis of dementia. It is useful for assessing deficits across multiple cognitive domains in a detailed manner. The resulting neuropsychological profile aids in differential diagnosis and formulation regarding what type of dementia is affecting a patient. In most cases it is not necessary to repeat a full neuropsychological battery later in the disease course as brief, less intensive assessments are adequate for tracking dementia. However, detailed neuropsychological outcomes may be useful in cases where further questions arise regarding the specific dementia profile displayed by the patient. Furthermore, while initial neuropsychological testing is mainly concerned with assessing deficits, later testing may be useful in assessing patient strengths, which may be called upon in developing an optimal treatment plan. The detailed information offered by a full battery of neuropsychological tests will also be important in assessing outcomes as improved cognition-sparing treatments are developed in the future. (The Tips and Tricks box includes the baseline neuropsychological battery recommended for the National Institute on Aging Consortium to Establish a Registry for Alzheimer's Disease.)

★ TIPS AND TRICKS

A number of dementia outcome instruments are available free in the public domain

- Montreal Cognitive Assessment: www. mocatest.org
- St. Louis University Mental Status Exam: http://medschool.slu.edu/ agingsuccessfully/pdfsurveys/ slumsexam_05.pdf
- Functional Assessment Questionnaire: www.alz.washington.edu/NONMEMBER/ UDS/DOCS/VER1_2/b7.pdf
- Quality of Life-AD: www.dementia-assessment.com.au/quality/QOL_handout_guidelines_scale.pdf
- Neuropsychiatric Inventory: http://npitest. net/
- Geriatric Depression Scale (Short Form): www.stanford.edu/~yesavage/GDS.english. short.html
- Zarit Burden Interview: www.aafp.org/ afp/2000/1215/p2613. html#afp20001215p2613-f1
- Revised Memory and Behavior Problem Checklist: www.alz.org/national/ documents/C_ASSESS-RevisedMemoryandBehCheck.pdf
- Clinical Dementia Rating Scale (free for individual and clinical use; training and resources): http://alzheimer.wustl.edu

Functional abilities

Functional abilities, including instrumental activities of daily living (IADLs) and activities of daily living (ADLs), are assessed along with cognition to determine dementia severity and stage. A patient's ability to independently carry out daily activities affects quality of life for both the patient and caregiver, and ultimately may determine whether costly institutionalization is needed. Furthermore, tracking functional outcomes is important in cases where there is potential for rehabilitation. There are numerous scales in existence to assess degree of disability and independence, but some have not been validated in dementia populations or include other domains in the assessment (i.e. behavioral problems), which may skew functional assessment.

The oldest and most widely used scales to assess functional ability are as follows.

Lawton Instrumental Activities of Daily Living Scale

This instrument assesses how a patient is functioning across eight domains, including using a telephone, shopping, food preparation, housekeeping, laundry, mode of transportation, responsibility for medications and ability to handle finances, providing an 8-point score with a higher score indicating better functioning and more independence. Traditionally, men were scored on only five of the domains, with housekeeping, food preparation, and laundry excluded. This is a brief and convenient scale, but has the disadvantage of relying on self- or caregiver report, which may lead to under- or overestimation of deficits.

The Katz Index of Independence in Activities of Daily Living

The Katz ADL ranks adequacy of performance in the six functions of bathing, dressing, toileting, transferring, continence, and feeding. It is scored from 0 to 6, with higher scores indicating better function. It is convenient and allows communication about function between providers, but has limited sensitivity to small degrees of change over time.

(Pfeffer) Functional Assessment Questionnaire (FAQ)

The FAQ consists of 10 items that assess functional activities including writing checks, paying bills, and keeping financial records; assembling tax or business records; shopping alone; playing games of skill; making coffee or tea; preparing a balanced meal; keeping track of current events; paying attention and understanding while reading or watching a TV show; remembering appointments, family occasions, and to take medications; and traveling out of the neighborhood or arranging transportation. Scores are based on information from an informant. Each element is scored on a scale from 0 (normal) to 3 (dependent). Overall scores range from 0 to 30 points, where higher scores indicate more functional impairment.

Quality of life

Over the past 20 years there has been a paradigm shift away from symptomatic medical treatment toward a more patient-focused model of care, in which overall well-being is paramount. This shift led to increased focus on quality of life (QoL), with resulting efforts to measure it in research and clinical practice. Lawton's model of QoL laid the groundwork for these scales by highlighting the multidimensional nature of QoL, requiring the need for both subjective and objective assessment of four main dimensions: behavioral competence, perceived QoL, psychological well-being, and environmental quality. What constitutes QoL continues to be a topic of debate, and attempts to quantify and measure a concept that is largely subjective and individual has led to a number of QoL rating instruments for various populations. Tailoring QoL measurements for assessment of dementia patients presents a specific set of issues to consider.

Quality of life in dementia is itself multifaceted and changes throughout the course of the disease. While patients with early dementia may experience high levels of autonomy related to their activities and environment, their psychological capacity, behavioral control, and environment may be drastically different in later stages. Many dementia QoL measures are stage specific for this reason. The ability of patients with progressive cognitive decline to accurately assess and report on their quality of life has also been questioned, leading to the use of caregiver report for a number of scales. Lastly, operational definitions of QoL in dementia can blur into other domains, such as function or neuropsychiatric symptoms. Clarification of which elements should be included in the potentially broad concept of QoL will be important for reliably tracking outcomes in this area. The following are a few of the most commonly used instruments for measuring QoL in dementia.

Alzheimer's Disease-Related Quality of Life (ADRQL)

The revised 40-item ADRQL assesses behaviors across five domains: social interaction (12 items), awareness of self (eight items), feelings and mood (12 items), enjoyment of activities (four items), and response to surroundings (four items). It involves a structured interview of a caregiver (formal or informal) by a trained interviewer or clinician. The overall score is determined as a percentage of 0 to 100, with higher scores reflecting higher quality of life. It was developed with the goal of assessing QoL response to therapeutic interventions for patients with AD across stages of disease and across various care settings.

Cornell-Brown Scale for QoL in Dementia (CBS)

The CBS is a 19-item scale developed on the premise that high QoL as it relates to dementia is indicated by the presence of positive affect, physical and psychological satisfaction, and self-esteem, and the relative absence of negative affect and experiences. It is administered by a clinician with combined input from both the patient and caregiver. Each item is scored from -2 to 2, with total scores of -38 to +38. Negative scores indicate poorer QoL and positive scores indicate better. Lower CBS QoL scores have been correlated with more severe dementia.

Quality of Life-Alzheimer's Disease (QoL-AD)

The QoL-AD consists of 13 items assessing mood, physical health, memory, relationships, self- esteem, and living situation. It uses combined information from both the patient and the caregiver, although they are assessed separately. Each item is rated on a four-point scale, with 1 being poor and 4 being excellent. Total scores range from 13 to 52. It generally takes about 15 min to administer, with the caregiver section requiring about 5 min and the patient section about 10 min to complete.

Neuropsychiatric symptoms

Neuropsychiatric symptoms are a defining characteristic of dementias, with up to 90% of dementia patients developing behavioral or psychological disturbance over the course of their illness. The symptoms experienced may include agitation, physical aggression, depression (with or without suicidal behavior), hallucinations, delusions, disinhibition and sexually inappropriate behavior, anxiety, apathy, and disturbances of appetite and sleep. Each dementia type has a typical neuropsychiatric symptom profile, but patients with any neurodegenerative illness may experience the range of symptoms. Furthermore, different symptoms may become more prominent at different stages of illness. To optimally address neuropsychiatric symptoms in dementia, they must be identified early and accurately, and outcomes should be followed over the course of the disease.

Assessing neuropsychiatric outcomes is instrumental in dementia care. These symptoms diminish quality of life for the patient and caregiver, increase financial costs and institutionalization, and worsen disease prognosis. Ongoing assessment is necessary in order to ensure safety and offer timely intervention. Patients experiencing neuropsychiatric symptoms should be seen routinely at least every 3–6 months, but more frequently in the setting of severe or dangerous symptoms and following changes in treatment. Inpatient psychiatric hospitalization should be considered in cases where the patient poses harm to themselves or those around them. The effect that neuropsychiatric symptoms have on caregivers should be considered in the assessment. A number of instruments have been developed to identify and track neuropsychiatric symptoms in dementia. Scales are available to conveniently assess global neuropsychiatric symptoms in dementia, as well as for tracking individual symptoms or sets of symptoms.

Neuropsychiatric Inventory (NPI)

The NPI is the instrument most widely used to assess global psychopathology in people with Alzheimer's disease and other dementias. It utilizes caregiver report to examine recent neuropsychiatric symptoms across 12 domains, including delusions, hallucinations, agitation, depression, anxiety, euphoria, apathy, disinhibition, irritability, aberrant behaviors, nighttime behaviors, and appetite changes. It provides scores for both symptom "frequency" and "severity," with a total resulting "frequency × severity" scores range from 0 to 144, with higher scores indicating greater psychopathology. It also incorporates a "distress" score to indicate how distressing a particular symptom is for the caregiver on a five-point scale. The NPI is useful in characterizing symptom profiles in specific neurodegenerative illness, and is sensitive to change in relation to treatment. As it was first developed to assess neuropsychiatric symptoms in the inpatient setting, it is clinically oriented. There is also an NPI-NH designed specifically to elicit information from formal caregivers in the nursing home setting and an NPI-Q version which is specifically used for assessing neuropsychiatric symptomatology in clinical practice settings. Both have been validated against the original NPI. The full version takes approximately 15 min to administer. It has the advantage of widespread use and has been translated into a number of languages.

Geriatric Depression Scale (GDS)

Depression is a common manifestation in nearly all forms of dementia. The GDS is a depression assessment tool commonly used in the clinical setting. The original form consists of 30 "yes" or "no" questions in reference to mood symptoms over the past week. A short version consisting of 15 questions has been developed and is now more common in clinical practice. The GDS is based on patient self-report, which limits utility in patients with moderate-to-severe dementia. However, its brevity and the simplicity of dichotomous answer choices make it easy to understand and administer to patients with mild-to-moderate dementia. Administration time for the short form is about 5–7 min. Scores of 0–4 are considered normal; 5–8 indicate mild depression; 9–11 indicate moderate depression; and 12–15 indicate severe depression. While the GDS is useful for screening and tracking depression symptoms, it is not a substitute for diagnostic interview by a mental health professional. It does not assess for suicidality.

Caregiver burden

Dementia affects not only individuals suffering from the illness but also the people caring for them. The majority of individuals with dementia are cared for at home by family members, with an estimated 15 million Americans providing unpaid care for a person with dementia. The concept of caregiver burden has come to encapsulate the emotional, physical, social, and financial burdens experienced by caregivers. Caregiver burden is high in those caring for dementia patients. As a group, caregivers experience higher levels of anxiety and depression, poorer physical health, and shortened life. Caregivers may become patients themselves because of the emotional and physical decline they experience, making caregiver distress a major public health issue. This distress continues even after a loved one with dementia is placed in a nursing facility, as many caregivers continue to provide emotional support and help with day-to-day care, as well as participating in medical, end-of-life and legal decision making. Interventions that lower caregiver distress have been shown to improve outcomes for caregivers themselves, as well as improving quality of life and delaying nursing home placement for those receiving care, all of which have major implications for healthcare costs and society.

The caregiving experience in dementia is complex and can be affected by a multitude of factors, including but not limited to depression and anxiety, cultural and ethnic background, other obligations of the caregiver (children, employment), the stage of the patient's dementia, family conflict, and the caregiver's own level of functioning. Efforts to incorporate interventions and track outcomes related to caregiver distress into clinical practice should take these factors into consideration. Available interventions typically consist of education, support groups, respite care, family therapy, individual therapy, or some combination of these. It is hoped that the development of new pharmacological treatments that slow or prevent cognitive deterioration will result in lower aggregate levels of caregiver burden over time. Various tools have been developed to assess and track levels of distress in those who care for individuals with dementia. It is important to utilize measures that incorporate psychological, physical, psychosocial, and financial aspects of caregiver burden into assessing outcomes.

Zarit Burden Interview

The Zarit Burden Interview was developed to measure subjective burden among caregivers of adults with dementia. The 22-item revised version is the instrument most widely used for assessment of caregiver burden in dementia research (the original version is 29 items and a short version is 12 items). It is completed by caregiver report. Each question is scored on a five-point scale from 0 (never) to 4 (nearly always present). Total scores range from 0 (low burden) to 88 (high burden). Items assess experiences regarding emotional state, health, finances, social life, and interpersonal relations.

Revised Memory and Behavior Problem Checklist (RMBPC)

The RMBPC consists of 24 caregiver report items inquiring about observable behavioral and memory problems in dementia patients and caregivers' reaction to these problems in the previous week. If the caregiver indicates that a particular problem has occurred, they then rate the degree of distress experienced due to the behavior on a five-point scale from 0 (not at all) to 4 (extremely). Scores range from 0 to 96, with higher total scores indicating greater behavioral burden. It provides a total score plus scores for three subscales: memory-related

problems, affective distress, and disruptive behaviors. The RMBPC has been validated for use with ethnically diverse caregivers in several studies.

Caregiver time-based assessments

One method for assessing caregiver burden is to utilize time spent on caregiving activities as a surrogate measure. Caregiver time includes time spent assisting an individual with dementia with IADLs, ADLs, behavioral problems, and other dementia-related needs. These scales have the advantage of quantifying the time requirements of caregiver burden in a way that allows the financial impact of both formal and informal caregiving activities to be calculated. Time-based methods are sensitive to change in cognitive function. Their disadvantages include a decreased ability to capture the subjective distress of the caregiver and dependence on caregiver recall for reporting, which may result in bias. An example of time-based caregiver burden scales is the Caregiver Activities Time Survey.

Global assessment

Global measures in dementia utilize information across domains to provide an overall impression of disease severity or to detect change in disease progression. Instruments for global dementia assessment are usually based on a semi-structured interview with the patient and a caregiver. They have the advantage of taking into account a breadth of information across domains, and unlike performance-based measures, these instruments provide information on clinically meaningful disease progression based on "real-world" outcomes. Global scales that assess severity of dementia provide a standard by which to communicate about a patient's dementia stage, but due to the heterogeneity among dementia patients, may not be particularly useful in appreciating effects of treatment or predicting illness course. On the other hand, a number of global dementia measures assess disease-related change. These scales are more useful for assessing response to treatment over time. Global assessments do not offer the sensitivity to small changes in specific domains provided by more specific assessments. Initial clinical global impression instruments were simple, unstructured scales that were found to inadequately detect treatment-related change. However, more structured, complex instruments have been developed over the past 20 years.

Clinical Dementia Rating Scale (CDR)

The CDR is a global assessment instrument that clinically stages the severity of cognitive-functional impairment in dementia. It involves a semi-structured interview with both patient and caregiver, with an estimated administration time of 40–75 min. It provides both a global score and a sum of boxes (SB) score. The global score uses an algorithm to transform ratings across six domains (memory, orientation, judgment and problem solving, community affairs, home and hobbies, and personal care) into a categorical staging of disease severity (none, questionable, mild, moderate, or severe). The SB score can range from 0 to 18 (0–3 points in each domain), with higher scores indicating greater impairment. More recently, it has been proposed that using the continuous CDR-SB scores to stage dementia severity offers advantages over using the global score, including easier calculation and increased precision in tracking changes over time. The amount of time required for administration of the CDR may be a disadvantage in the clinical setting.

Alzheimer's Disease Cooperative Study-Clinical Global Impression of Change (ADCS-CGIC)

The ADCS-CGIC is a seven-point categorical scale that provides a single global rating of change from baseline. It utilizes both direct observation of the patient and interview of an informant in order to observe change in the patient's cognitive, functional, and behavioral performance. Scores range from 1 to 7, with a score of 1 indicating marked improvement, a score of 7 marked worsening, and a score of 4 no change. As with other CGI scales, an overarching assumption is that the rater is a skilled clinician.

Hospitalizations, Nursing Home Placement, and Mortality

The number of people with Alzheimer's disease and other dementias will continue to grow as the world's population ages, with an estimated 115 million people expected to have Alzheimer's disease by 2050. This presents a major public health concern given the increased morbidity associated with dementia. The total cost of caring for patients with Alzheimer's disease in the US in 2011 was $183 billion, and it has been estimated that caring for patients with Alzheimer's disease costs Medicare 60% more than

SCIENCE REVISITED

Potential modifiers of rate of cognitive decline in Alzheimer's disease

Factor	Rate of cognitive decline
• More severe cognitive impairment at baseline	Increase
• Younger age of onset	Increase
• Vascular risk factors	Generally increase
• Focal neurological/ motor signs	Increase
• Apathy	Increase
• Very total high tau and ptau	Increase
• Very low Abeta1-42 level	Increase
• Sex	Mixed (increased rates shown for both males and females in different studies)
• Diabetes mellitus	Mixed (both increased and decreased rates shown)
• High educational level	Mixed
• APOE 4	Mixed (controversial)

treating those without dementia. The increased costs to society and the increased suffering experienced by dementia patients make working to improve outcomes in terms of hospitalizations and nursing home placement a crucial pursuit in healthcare. While tracking these outcomes is generally done through large epidemiological studies, reviewing the current knowledge about morbidity and mortality outcomes in dementia provides perspective on how quality improvements in the domains discussed earlier in the chapter may also improve "downstream" outcomes related to hospitalization, nursing home placement, and mortality.

People with dementia experience increased rates of hospitalization and poorer outcomes when hospitalized. Demented patients are at increased risk of admission for a number of conditions, including those for which proactive primary care might prevent hospitalization (i.e. pneumonia, congestive heart failure, urinary tract infections, dehydration, etc.). The reasons for increased hospitalization in this population are multifactorial, but include increased morbidity related to the cause of dementia itself (i.e. stroke), conditions resulting from dementia (i.e. swallowing difficulties and increased risk of aspiration), and increased difficulty treating co-morbid conditions due to the patient's cognitive impairment. Cognitive impairment may lead to delay in treatment because of a patient's inability to report symptoms, and functional decline may make treating other conditions challenging, for example if the patient is unable to take medications properly. Clinician thresholds for hospitalizing demented patients may also be lower. Furthermore, patients may be admitted or visit the emergency room more often for neuropsychiatric disturbances.

Once in the hospital, demented patients are at increased risk for further cognitive and functional decline, delirium, and iatrogenic complications. Tracking outcomes and examining the reasons for increased hospitalization of dementia patients may lead to the development of preventive strategies to ameliorate hospitalization risk in the outpatient setting.

Dementia makes placement in a nursing home more likely and shortens life expectancy. Nursing home placement has been associated with specific patient characteristics, including living alone, greater functional impairment, more severe cognitive deficits, and higher levels of behavioral symptoms. In contrast, some characteristics, such as black or Hispanic ethnicity, have been associated with lower rates of nursing placement. Individuals with dementia are more likely to be placed in a care facility when their caregivers are older, less functional, and experience higher levels of caregiver burden. Estimates of survival from time of dementia onset typically range from 5 to 10 years, although there is heterogeneity between types of dementia as well as within a specific diagnosis. Factors including poorer cognitive and functional status, medical co-morbidities, and extrapyramidal symptoms are associated with shorter life expectancy in dementia. Men with dementia generally have shorter life expectancies than women. Survival estimates have been less than 5 years when including patients with rapidly progressive dementias. Based on these predictors, tracking and improving upon outcomes related to function, behavior and caregiver burden may ultimately delay nursing home placement, improve survival, and decrease related financial and societal costs.

More on pay for performance and quality measures

The Institute of Medicine (IOM) proposes that quality healthcare should be safe, effective, patient centered, timely, efficient, and equitable. Pay for performance programs utilize specific quality of care measures to assess the performance of healthcare providers compared to preset standards. In the US, the increasing strain of healthcare expenditures has led Medicare and insurance companies to begin implementing pay for performance programs, which ideally promote reduced costs, improved access, and increased quality of services. However, it is not entirely clear how such programs may affect healthcare provision, especially in specialized areas such as dementia care.

The American Academy of Neurology (AAN) position on pay for performance emphasizes the need for these programs to focus on quality care and patient safety over efficiency and cutting costs. It also highlights a number of potential barriers to neurologist participation should these programs not be implemented in a thoughtful and careful manner: costs of documentation, difficulties with providing sufficient data in specialty practices, and the possibility that these programs will encourage diagnostic tests over thoughtful and skilled patient care. Prior to implementation, it will be important for providers of dementia care to develop their own important, valid, and practical quality outcome measures. This chapter is an effort to take a step in the process.

A number of programs for reporting on quality measures have already been put into place. The Physician Quality Reporting Initiative (PQRI) first started in 2007 with a 6-month voluntary reporting period. In 2011 the program became known as the Physician Quality Reporting System (PQRS). Each year the Center for Medicare and Medicaid Services (CMS) puts out a call for measures to be submitted to the program and each year new measures are accepted. These measures are ideally evidence based and are often drawn from clinical guidelines. An example from 2011 is "Measure #150: Back Pain: Advice for Normal Activities." If this information was given and documented this could be reported.

Currently there are four ways to report measures; via claims, a qualified electronic health record (EHR), a registry or a group. Each reporting system has a different list of measures. The reportable measures if done via claims are determined by looking at the ICD-9 and CPT codes. You must report at least 50% of all eligible patients for a given measure to reach the threshold for the incentive. For EHR reporting, there are currently approximately 50–60 measures. Registry reporting involves partnering with a CMS-qualified registry which reports to the CMS on the participants' behalf. There is often a cost involved for this process. There are also group reporting options for groups of 20 or more. There are 29 group measures mostly related to general practice.

Currently some measures, such as those related to Parkinson's disease, dementia, and sleep apnea, are only reportable via a registry. Other neurology measures such as those for epilepsy can be reported via claims or a qualified registry. In 2001 proper reporting of the PQRS could have resulted in an incentive payment of 1% of total Medicare Physician Fee Schedule (MPFS) allowed charges for Medicare and 0.5% for Medicaid. This percentage decreases each year until 2015 when it becomes a mandatory program. At that time there will be a 1.5% penalty on Medicare charges and in 2016 and beyond it increases to a 2% penalty. The American Academy of Neurology is an excellent resource for following comment periods and specifics of implementation through their website, undertaking educational sessions offered at annual meetings and seeking help from their performance measurement staff.

Practical approach to capturing key outcomes

Most work related to dementia outcomes has been for the purpose of clinical trials; using instruments in the clinical setting requires further considerations. While validity and reliability are intrinsically important to rating instruments in general, convenience and practicality become central issues when using them in the clinical realm. Factors including administration time, distress and fatigue for the patient and caregiver, use of clinical resources, and an ability to easily collect and track outcomes data should be taken into account. If well thought out, incorporating outcomes measures into clinical practice can seamlessly supplement sound clinical judgment and enhance the clinician–patient relationship. They also may serve as a means to meet the PQRS requirements detailed above.

Assessments need to be tailored to the cognitive and functional capacity of many dementia patients (and potentially their caregivers) to prevent everyone from being overwhelmed. The timing and setting of assessments can be arranged to minimize fatigue. Scales assessing neuropsychiatric symptoms, caregiver burden, and QoL can be filled out prior to coming in for a scheduled appointment. Likewise, caregivers can fill out questionnaires in a separate area while the cognitive assessment and physical exam are being performed with the patient. Certain domains, such as caregiver distress and QoL, may be evaluated by various members of the care team, such as social workers or nurses. Having a routine plan for when and how assessments are performed is crucial to ensure that consistent, complete data are collected at each visit. Following collection, outcomes data should be amassed in a central location. Electronic medical records can be utilized with preset forms allowing for easy input, tracking and even analysis over time.

Considering these practical factors as outcomes assessments are incorporated into clinical practice will minimize administrative problems and smooth the transition as regulatory and reimbursement agencies require these measures to be reported.

Conclusion

Tracking outcomes in dementia care has important implications for patients, their families, and society. Comprehensive dementia care requires assessing outcomes across a number of domains, including cognition, functional disability, QoL, neuropsychiatric symptoms, and caregiver distress. Assessing dementia-related outcomes across domains allows clinicians to better appreciate the clinical course of dementia and to evaluate the impact of interventions. It will also inform future research, foster communication in the field, and promote best practice. Improving dementia outcomes across clinical domains has the potential to decrease the morbidity, mortality, and financial impact related to dementia as the world's population ages. There are currently a number of convenient, valid, and reliable outcomes instruments available that can be incorporated into clinical practice. The UDS recommended assessment battery is an example of a standardized set of assessments that can be used to track outcomes across institutions and can serve as a springboard for future work in this area. Available instruments each have strengths and weaknesses, and future endeavors should focus on developing valid, reliable, and convenient instruments that can be used in the clinical setting and are sensitive to change across stages of dementia severity. Pay for performance programs base reimbursement on outcomes, and will likely become the norm in years to come.

Ultimately, utilizing outcomes measures in the clinical setting serves the purpose of improving the quality of care provided to dementia patients and their families.

Further reading

Cummings JL. The Neuropsychiatric Inventory: assessing psychopathology in dementia patients. *Neurology* 1997; **48**(5 Suppl 6): S10–16.

Davis KL, Marin DB, Kane R, et al. The Caregiver Activity Survey (CAS): development and validation of a new measure for caregivers of persons with Alzheimer's disease. *Int J Geriatr Psychiatry* 1997; **12**(10): 978–88.

Folstein MF, Folstein SE, McHugh PR. "Mini-mental state". A practical method for grading the cognitive state of patients for the clinician. *J Psychiatr Res* 1975; **12**(3): 189–98.

Hughes CP, Berg L, Danziger WL, Coben LA, Martin RL. A new clinical scale for the staging of dementia. *Br J Psychiatry* 1982; **140**: 566–72.

Katz S, Ford AB, Moskowitz RW, Jackson BA, Jaffe MW. Studies of illness in the aged. The Index of ADL: a standardized measure of biological and psychosocial function. *JAMA* 1963; **185**: 914–19.

Lawton MP, Brody EM. Assessment of older people: self-maintaining and instrumental activities of daily living. *Gerontologist* 1969; **9**(3): 179–86.

Logsdon RG, Gibbons LE, McCurry SM, Teri L. Assessing quality of life in older adults with cognitive impairment. *Psychosom Med* 2002; **64**(3): 510–19.

Morris JC, Weintraub S, Chui HC, et al. The Uniform Data Set (UDS): clinical and cognitive variables and descriptive data from Alzheimer Disease Centers. *Alzheimer Dis Assoc Disord* 2006; **20**(4): 210–16.

Nasreddine ZS, Phillips NA, Bedirian V, et al. The Montreal Cognitive Assessment, MoCA: a brief screening tool for mild cognitive impairment. *J Am Geriatr Soc* 2005; **53**(4): 695–9.

Pfeffer RI, Kurosaki TT, Harrah CH Jr, Chance JM, Filos S. Measurement of functional activities in older adults in the community. *J Gerontol* 1982; **37**(3): 323–9.

Rabins PV, Kasper JD, Kleinman L, Black BS, Patrick DL. Concepts and methods in development of the ADRQL: an instrument for assessing health-related quality of life in persons with Alzheimer's disease. *J Ment Health Aging* 1999; **15**: 33–48.

Ready RE, Ott BR, Grace J, Fernandez I. The Cornell-Brown Scale for Quality of Life in dementia. *Alzheimer Dis Assoc Disord* 2002; **16**(2): 109–15.

Rosen WG, Mohs RC, Davis KL. A new rating scale for Alzheimer's disease. *Am J Psychiatry* 1984; **141**(11): 1356–64.

Schneider LS, Olin JT, Doody RS, et al. Validity and reliability of the Alzheimer's Disease Cooperative Study-Clinical Global Impression of Change. The Alzheimer's Disease Cooperative Study. *Alzheimer Dis Assoc Disord* 1997; **11**(Suppl 2): S22–32.

Tariq SH, Tumosa N, Chibnall JT, Perry MH 3rd, Morley JE. Comparison of the Saint Louis University mental status examination and the mini-mental state examination for detecting dementia and mild neurocognitive disorder – a pilot study. *Am J Geriatr Psychiatry* 2006; **14**(11): 900–10.

Teri L, Truax P, Logsdon R, Uomoto J, Zarit S, Vitaliano PP. Assessment of behavioral problems in dementia: the Revised Memory and Behavior Problems Checklist. *Psychol Aging* 1992; **7**(4): 622–31.

Yesavage JA, Brink TL, Rose TL, et al. Development and validation of a geriatric depression screening scale: a preliminary report. *J Psychiatr Res* 1982–1983; **17**(1): 37–49.

Zarit SH, Todd PA, Zarit JM. Subjective burden of husbands and wives as caregivers: a longitudinal study. *Gerontologist* 1986; **26**(3): 260–6.

12

Primary Prevention of Dementia

Joseph Quinn

Oregon Health and Science University and Portland VA Medical Center, USA

Introduction

It is almost predictable, when a dementia patient is accompanied by adult children, that neurologists will be asked by non-demented family members, "What do I need to do to avoid getting dementia myself?" Typically this is a "door-knob" question, meaning that it comes as the clinician is grasping the knob of the examining room door, thinking the visit is over. The question also comes from peers at continuing medical education (CME) conferences, from friends and family at social events, and basically from everyone who has gotten old enough to start worrying about Alzheimer's disease. It consequently deserves a chapter of its own, even though at present we cannot point to established practice parameters for the prevention of Alzheimer's disease or dementia.

In April 2010 the National Institutes of Health convened a consensus conference in an effort to develop an evidence-based statement about how best to slow cognitive decline with aging and prevent late-life dementia. The facts were reviewed with 2 days of expert testimony, looking at the available evidence on nutrition, mental exercise, physical exercise, vascular risk factor control, and other pertinent topics. An impartial panel of experts then reviewed the data and delivered their conclusion that despite an abundance of risk factors and an abundance of research, no intervention has been shown to be effective for slowing the rate of cognitive decline or dementia.

> ### ⚖ SCIENCE REVISITED
>
> The NIH State of the Science Conference statement on Preventing Alzheimer's Disease and Cognitive Decline is available in its entirety at http://consensus.nih.gov/2010/alz.htm. From the abstract: "Currently, firm conclusions cannot be drawn about the association of any modifiable risk factor with cognitive decline of Alzheimer's disease ... Evidence is insufficient to support the use of pharmaceutical agents or dietary supplements to prevent cognitive decline of Alzheimer's disease."

Obviously this is not a satisfying answer for clinicians or patients, and it is important to emphasize that the panel did not conclude that risk factor modification has been proven ineffective. For a variety of reasons, many important risk factors have not been "put to the test" in a controlled clinical trial. The challenge for clinicians is to find a practical course between false claims and therapeutic nihilism in making recommendations for cognitive health. We will attempt to chart such a course here by reviewing relevant risk factors, then reviewing completed clinical trials attempting to modify these risk factors, then reviewing published projections of the benefits of risk factor modification, and finally concluding with recommendations that are practical, concrete, and inarguably beneficial for general health even if unproven for cognitive health.

Alzheimer's disease and vascular risk

In considering the prominence of vascular risk factors in the following list of dementia risk factors, it is important to remember that all large risk factor studies rely on clinical, rather than pathological, diagnosis of Alzheimer's disease, and even pathologically confirmed Alzheimer's disease includes some degree of concomitant cerebrovascular disease. In fact, several studies have emphasized that concomitant cerebrovascular disease increases the likelihood of "clinical expression" of dementia. In other words, risk factors for Alzheimer's disease (AD) are not necessarily risk factors for Alzheimer-specific lesions like plaques and tangles, but may include risk factors for subclinical cerebrovascular disease, which in turn modifies the expression of AD.

What are the best established modifiable risk factors for Alzheimer's dementia?

Hypertension

Several systematic reviews have found that the effect of hypertension upon dementia risk appears to be age dependent. Midlife hypertension consistently increases the risk of late-life dementia, while the effect of late-life hypertension upon dementia risk is less clear, possibly because of the confounding effects of medication and iatrogenic hypotension. Pooled results from systematic studies yielded a relative risk of 1.61 for AD among subjects with midlife hypertension.

Smoking

Although some early studies surprisingly found a reduced incidence of dementia in smokers, more recent longitudinal studies have consistently found an increased incidence of dementia in smokers. The most comprehensive metaanalysis to date found a relative risk of 1.59 for AD among active smokers.

Depression

Depression has consistently been identified as a risk factor for Alzheimer's and dementia, with some studies finding that onset of first depression in later life carries the strongest risk of dementia. Two recent metaanalyses have found that any history of depression is associated with a two-fold increase in the risk of Alzheimer's disease or dementia with relative risks ranging from 1.87 to 2.03.

Physical inactivity

One systematic review of physical inactivity and cognitive function observed that 20 out of 24 longitudinal studies found that physical inactivity was associated with some level of cognitive impairment. A second systematic review examined the association between physical inactivity and dementia in 16 studies, and found a relative risk for all-cause dementia of 1.39 and for Alzheimer's disease of 1.82 in the most physically inactive individuals compared to the most active.

Cognitive inactivity

Although it is intuitive to think that cognitive exercise is critical to brain health, the variables are much more difficult to quantify in this area and the literature is consequently more limited. However, one systematic analysis compared dementia risk in subjects according to whether or not they engaged in "cognitively stimulating leisure activities" and found that subjects who engaged in such activities had a reduced risk of dementia, with an estimated relative risk of 0.5.

Dietary factors

Obesity

There appears to be a parallel between obesity and hypertension in terms of the effects of age upon risk factor modification. As with hypertension, studies of midlife obesity consistently find an increased risk of Alzheimer's disease in obese subjects with a relative risk estimated at 1.59, while late-life obesity does not appear to be a robust risk factor. In this case, the *post facto* explanation is that early disease-associated weight loss masks the effect of obesity upon brain health in late life.

Diabetes mellitus

Diabetes mellitus has been associated with an increased risk of dementia in several studies. One metaanalysis of nine prospective studies found a relative risk of AD of 1.39 and all-cause dementia of 1.47 in diabetics, while a second metaanalysis of eight prospective studies found a relative risk of 1.54 for all-cause dementia in diabetics.

Hypercholesterolemia

Several studies have reported an increased risk of Alzheimer's disease and all-cause dementia in patients with hypercholesterolemia. There is some evidence from animal models and cerebrospinal fluid (CSF) biomarker studies to indicate that statins may have effects on AD pathology rather than on concomitant vascular pathology, but clinical trials have been disappointing to date.

Low omega 3 fatty acid intake

Some (but not all) population-based studies have shown a reduced risk of AD in individuals who consume higher levels of fish, which are rich in the omega 3 fatty acids eicosapentaenoic acid (EPA) and docosahexaenoic acid (DHA), the latter of which is the most abundant polyunsaturated fatty acid (PUFA) in the brain. Animal studies have suggested that DHA intake modifies AD pathology, but clinical trials have been disappointing.

Low antioxidant intake

Several risk factor studies have provided evidence that consumption of vitamin E, vitamin C, or the combination is associated with a reduced risk of AD. As with statins and omega 3s, however, clinical trials have been discouraging to date.

B vitamin-related hyperhomocysteinemia

Elevated serum homocysteine, which in many cases is a reflection of B vitamin status, has been associated with increased risk of stroke, dementia, and AD. Trials of B vitamins for the treatment or prevention of AD have shown successful reduction of serum homocysteine, but mixed effects on cognitive outcomes.

Trace metals

Patients and family members continue to ask about the effects of environmental aluminum upon AD risk since this was reported in the 1970s, but research on this topic has not borne out the "aluminum hypothesis" and most people in the field no longer consider aluminum a relevant factor.

However, some more recent evidence has implicated copper intake in the pathogenesis of AD, with both epidemiological and animal studies suggesting an interaction between dietary copper and dietary lipids.

Medications

Non-steroidal antiinflammatory drug usage

More than 20 studies of the effect of NSAID use upon dementia risk have concluded that NSAID users have a lower risk of Alzheimer's dementia compared to non-users. The remarkable consistency of this epidemiological finding has led to controlled clinical trials which will be discussed in the next section.

Estrogen

It is difficult to believe that as recently as the late 1990s, review articles were concluding that estrogen replacement therapy at menopause had great potential for the prevention of AD. The opinion regarding estrogen for dementia prevention has since been dramatically reversed on the basis of clinical trials. Interestingly, investigators in this area are now postulating that there may be a "critical period" for estrogen use in midlife, so that estrogen may be a third dementia risk factor which cannot be fully appreciated without careful consideration of interactions with age of exposure.

What modifiable risk factors have been evaluated in controlled clinical trials?

Many clinical trials have been designed and conducted on the basis of the flawed hypothesis that the pathogenic mechanisms which initiate AD continue to operate after dementia is manifest. In other words, many clinical trials based on the risk factor data just described tested the hypothesis that risk factor modification would slow the rate of progression of established AD, rather than testing whether risk factor modification would prevent AD. The reasons for this phenomenon are practical: trials to slow the rate of progression of AD require far fewer subjects, shorter periods of observation, and less money than prevention studies.

> **✋ CAUTION**
>
> Extrapolating from epidemiological studies to clinical practice is dangerous.
>
> Clinical trials of estrogen and NSAIDs, for example, have shown intolerable levels of morbidity, even beyond the known risks of thrombosis with estrogen and gastrointestinal bleeding with NSAIDs. Since there are no proven methods for reducing dementia risk, any risk factor modification recommendations need to consider all aspects of an individual's health, and should be confined to recommendations that are known to have significant health benefits.

One partial solution to this conundrum is to conduct prevention studies in individuals with 'pre-Alzheimer's disease" which is currently operationalized as "mild cognitive impairment" (MCI). However, it should be emphasized that an intervention's failure to alter the natural history of AD or MCI does not preclude the possibility that the same intervention could have an effective role in the primary prevention of AD. The reality, however, is that enthusiasm for targeting a given risk factor is greatly reduced by any negative clinical trial, so many of these risk factors have been abandoned after negative trials in AD. The following discussion of risk factor modification trials will distinguish trials in AD and MCI from primary prevention trials.

As shown in Table 12.1, very few randomized, placebo-controlled dementia prevention trials of risk factor modification have been performed. Many are precluded by ethical considerations, such as trials of blood pressure control and depression treatment, as it is not acceptable to withhold effective therapy for the sake of proving a scientific point. Several risk factors (e.g. statins, omega 3 fatty acids, antioxidants, B vitamins, NSAIDs, estrogens) have been systematically modified in randomized placebo-controlled trials to slow the progression of AD and all have failed. A smaller number of risk factors (NSAIDs, antioxidants, B vitamins) have been evaluated in MCI subjects. While there were some encouraging results with B vitamins slowing rates of cognitive decline and brain atrophy, none of these interventions has been shown to prevent progression of MCI to dementia.

Primary prevention trials have been conducted with hormone replacement, with NSAIDs, and with *Ginkgo biloba*. The Women's Health Initiative Memory Study (WHIMS) tested the hypothesis that estrogen replacement would reduce the incidence of dementia in postmenopausal women. However, just the opposite was observed relatively early in the study: women receiving estrogen supplements had a higher rate of dementia compared to those who received placebo. In many ways this study should serve as a cautionary tale for clinicians who would like to extrapolate from epidemiology to clinical practice. There is a real risk of doing harm in the absence of definitive evidence for a particular intervention, particularly in the area of preventive therapy in healthy individuals, where the tolerance for morbidity is lower than in the treatment of symptomatic subjects.

The experience with NSAIDs for AD prevention is similar. The Alzheimer's Disease Antiinflammatory Prevention Trial (ADAPT) tested the hypothesis that naproxen or the COX-2 selective NSAID celecoxib would reduce the incidence of dementia in subjects at risk because of age and family history. The treatment arms of ADAPT were terminated prematurely by the Data Safety and Monitoring Board because of excessive morbidity in the NSAID-treated arms. Some *post hoc* analyses have been completed, but the primary hypothesis regarding dementia outcomes remains essentially untested.

A primary prevention study of *Ginkgo biloba* extract represents the only large primary prevention study which has been completed without excess morbidity in the treatment arm, but unfortunately this good tolerability was not accompanied by clinical efficacy. The Ginkgo Evaluation of Memory (GEM) study tested the hypothesis that *Ginkgo biloba* extract would reduce the incidence of dementia, based in part on ginkgo's established antioxidant effects. After a median of 6 years of follow-up, the authors concluded that *Ginkgo biloba* extract was not effective at reducing cognitive decline or the incidence of dementia.

A 2009 Cochrane analysis of statins for the prevention of dementia concluded that there is no evidence for a dementia-preventive effect of statin therapy based on two large trials: HSP 2002 and PROSPER. However, it should be emphasized that neither of those trials was specifically designed for detecting dementia prevention effects; cognitive and functional assessments were added on to these cardiovascular studies. While it is true that no cognitive benefits of statin therapy were appreciated in the 3–5 years of follow-up in these two large trials, this does not preclude the possibility of long-term cognitive benefits from judicious application of statins according to established lipid-lowering guidelines.

The conclusions of the NIH Dementia Prevention consensus conference may appear more understandable after review of these dismal findings, but before concluding that there is nothing to recommend to individuals at risk, we will return to consideration of those risk factors in Table 12.1 which cannot be ethically studied in a placebo-controlled manner.

Table 12.1 Randomized clinical trials of dementia risk factor modification

Dementia risk factor	Alzheimer's disease	Mild cognitive impairment	Primary prevention of dementia	Cognitive effects in healthy elderly
Hypertension	Placebo control unethical	Placebo control unethical	Placebo control unethical	Placebo control unethical
Smoking	Placebo control unethical	Placebo control unethical	Placebo control unethical	Placebo control unethical
Depression	Placebo control unethical	Placebo control unethical	Placebo control unethical	Placebo control unethical
Physical inactivity	No studies identified	No studies identified	No studies identified	Improved executive function
Cognitive inactivity	No studies identified	No studies identified	No studies identified	Domain-specific improvements
Obesity	Placebo control unethical	Placebo control unethical	Placebo control unethical	Placebo control unethical
Diabetes mellitus	Placebo control unethical*	Placebo control unethical	Placebo control unethical	Placebo control unethical*
Hypercholesterolemia	Statins failed (in AD patients who did not meet standard lipid-lowering criteria)	No studies identified	No evidence of effect on dementia in HPS 2002	No effect on cognition in PROSPER or HPS 2002
Omega 3 fatty acids	Mixed omega 3s and DHA alone failed	No studies identified	No studies identified	Post hoc analysis showed effect on memory
Antioxidants	Vitamin E failed	Vitamin E failed	Ginkgo failed to prevent dementia (GEMS)	No studies identified
Homocysteine-lowering B vitamins	B vitamins failed	Slowed cognitive decline and brain atrophy (VITACOG)	No studies identified	Folic acid effective
Copper lowering	No studies identified	No studies identified	No studies identified	No studies identified
Non-steroidal antiinflammatory drugs	Naproxen and rofecoxib failed	Rofexocib failed	ADAPT prematurely terminated due to morbidity of NSAIDs	No studies identified
Estrogen	Failed × 2	No studies identified	Increased risk of dementia in WHIMS	No benefit

AD, Alzheimer's disease; DHA, docosohexaenoic acid.

Is there a way to evaluate the cognitive benefits of controlling depression and established vascular risk factors?

Not long after the NIH issued its pessimistic statement about dementia prevention, an analysis of the potential benefit of treating the "untestable" risk factors was published in *Lancet Neurology* by Barnes and Yaffe. The authors reviewed the literature to define the relative risks associated with each of these factors, then defined the prevalence of each risk factor, and finally calculated the effect upon AD prevalence achieved by reducing each risk factor by 10% or 25%. They conclude that a 10% reduction in all seven risk factors could prevent 1.1 million AD cases worldwide and 184,000 AD cases in the US, while a 25% reduction of all seven risk factors could prevent 3 million AD cases worldwide and 492,000 cases in the US. While these numbers are based on assumptions rather than on clinical trial data, the recommendation for modifying these particular risk factors for the sake of general health is inarguable – it is already the standard of care to do so.

How can these recommendations be translated into concrete and professionally responsible advice for subjects at risk?

In order for such advice to be practical, it has to be concrete and specific. In order for it to be professionally responsible, it should be reviewed and vetted in a rigorous fashion by appropriate medical experts. With respect to vascular risk factors, a user-friendly program of recommendations has recently been composed by the American Heart Association/American Stroke Association (AHA/ASA). While these recommendations are aimed at cardiovascular disease and stroke rather than at cognitive function *per se*, clinicians can be comfortable that the guidelines have been carefully reviewed before release and promotion. The program initiated in 2010 is called "Life's Simple 7" and provides specific guidelines for controlling most of the same risk factors analyzed by Barnes and Yaffe.

1) Physical activity: aim for 150 min per week of vigorous exercise.
2) Control cholesterol: aim for total cholesterol < 200 mg/dL.
3) Healthy diet: aim for compliance with elements of the AHA diet (vegetables and fruits, fiber-rich wholegrain foods, fish twice a week, cut back on saturated and trans fats, cholesterol, and added sugars).
4) Hypertension: aim for ≤ 120/80.
5) Control weight: aim for BMI < 25.
6) Control blood glucose: aim for fasting glucose < 100
7) Stop smoking.

A common response to this type of advice is "Of course, I already know all that and do my best." But the AHA points out that *less than 2%* of Americans actually meet these simple recommendations, so there is much work to be done in terms of education and promotion of vascular health.

> ### ★ TIPS AND TRICKS
>
> Refer family members to patient-friendly websites for responsible advice on dementia prevention.
>
> - Alzheimer's Association: www.alz.org/research/science/alzheimers_prevention_and_risk.asp
> - American Heart Association/American Stroke Association: www.heart.org
> - "Life's Simple 7" patient-friendly site for practical, safe tips for vascular risk factor management: http://mylifecheck.heart.org

A final word

Another modifiable risk factor for AD is low educational attainment, which has not been emphasized here because the goal is to provide responsible advice to adults. However, the late Dr William Markesbery, a national leader in AD research, was fond of concluding lectures to laypeople by making the points that educational attainment is a well-established means of reducing the risk of Alzheimer's disease, and one of the greatest determinants of educational attainment is whether parents read to their children. So, as Dr Markesbery used to say in dismissing his audience at the end of his lectures, "If you really want to reduce the incidence of Alzheimer's disease, then you should all go home now and read to your kids."

Further reading

Barnes DE, Yaffe K. The projected effect of risk factor reduction on Alzheimer's disease prevalence. *Lancet Neurol* 2011; **10**(9): 819–28.

Daviglus ML, Bell CC, Berrettini W, et al. National Institutes of Health State-of-the-Science Conference statement: preventing Alzheimer disease and cognitive decline. *Ann Intern Med* 2010; **153**(3): 176–81.

DeKosky ST, Williamson JD, Fitzpatrick AL, et al. Ginkgo biloba for prevention of dementia: a randomized controlled trial. *JAMA* 2008; **300**(19): 2253–62.

de Jager CA, Oulhaj A, Jacoby R, Refsum H, Smith AD. Cognitive and clinical outcomes of homocysteine-lowering B-vitamin treatment in mild cognitive impairment: a randomized controlled trial. *Int J Geriatr Psychiatry* 2012; **27**(6): 592–600.

Lyketsos CG, Breitner JC, Green RC, et al. Naproxen and celecoxib do not prevent AD in early results from a randomized controlled trial. *Neurology* 2007; **68**(21): 1800–8.

McGuinness B, Craig D, Bullock R, Passmore P. Statins for the prevention of dementia. *Cochrane Database Syst Rev* 2009; **2**: CD003160.

Morris MC, Evans DA, Tangney CC, et al. Dietary copper and high saturated and trans fat intakes associated with cognitive decline. *Arch Neurol* 2006; **63**(8): 1085–8.

Patterson C, Feightner JW, Garcia A, Hsiung GY, MacKnight C, Sadovnick AD. Diagnosis and treatment of dementia: 1. Risk assessment and primary prevention of Alzheimer disease. *Can Med Assoc J* 2008; **178**(5): 548–56.

Shumaker SA, Legault C, Rapp SR, et al. Estrogen plus progestin and the incidence of dementia and mild cognitive impairment in postmenopausal women: the Women's Health Initiative Memory Study: a randomized controlled trial. *JAMA* 2003; **289**(20): 2651–62.

Smith AD, Smith SM, de Jager CA, et al. Homocysteine-lowering by B vitamins slows the rate of accelerated brain atrophy in mild cognitive impairment: a randomized controlled trial. *PLoS One* 2010; **5**(9): e12244.

Index

Note: Page numbers in *italics* refer to Figures; those in **bold** to Tables.